INTEGRATIVE
HYPNOTHERAPY

Commissioning Editor: Claire Wilson
Development Editor: Natalie Meylan, Louisa Welch
Project Manager: Sukanthi Sukumar
Designer: Kirsteen Wright
Illustration Manager: Bruce Hogarth

INTEGRATIVE HYPNOTHERAPY
COMPLEMENTARY APPROACHES IN CLINICAL CARE

Edited by

Anne Cawthorn MSc, BSc (Hons), RGN, RNT, Dip Nursing, Dip Hypno, UKCP Reg, MIFPA
Macmillan Living Well Specialist Practitioner
The Living Well Centre
Blythe House Hospice
High Peak, Derbyshire, UK

Peter A. Mackereth PhD, MA, RGN, Dip Nursing, Cert Ed
Clinical Lead
Complementary Therapies and Smoking Cessation
The Christie NHS Foundation Trust
Manchester, UK

Forewords by
Aaron Kenneth Ward-Atherton
Lord of Witley & Hurcott Worcestershire
Patron of the Complementary Therapies Department
The Christie NHS Foundation Trust, Manchester, UK

Bernadette Hillon
Patient

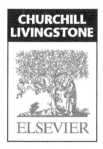

CHURCHILL
LIVINGSTONE

ELSEVIER

Edinburgh   London   New York   Oxford   Philadelphia   St Louis   Sydney   Toronto   2010

CHURCHILL
LIVINGSTONE
ELSEVIER

ISBN 978-0-7020-3082-6

British Library Cataloguing in Publication Data
A catalogue record for this book is available from the British Library

Library of Congress Cataloging in Publication Data
A catalog record for this book is available from the Library of Congress

Notices

Knowledge and best practice in this field are constantly changing. As new research and experience broaden our understanding, changes in research methods, professional practices, or medical treatment may become necessary.

Practitioners and researchers must always rely on their own experience and knowledge in evaluating and using any information, methods, compounds, or experiments described herein. In using such information or methods they should be mindful of their own safety and the safety of others, including parties for whom they have a professional responsibility.

With respect to any drug or pharmaceutical products identified, readers are advised to check the most current information provided (i) on procedures featured or (ii) by the manufacturer of each product to be administered, to verify the recommended dose or formula, the method and duration of administration, and contraindications. It is the responsibility of practitioners, relying on their own experience and knowledge of their patients, to make diagnoses, to determine dosages and the best treatment for each individual patient, and to take all appropriate safety precautions.

To the fullest extent of the law, neither the Publisher nor the authors, contributors, or editors, assume any liability for any injury and/or damage to persons or property as a matter of products liability, negligence or otherwise, or from any use or operation of any methods, products, instructions, or ideas contained in the material herein.

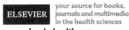
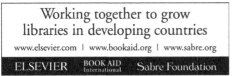

CONTENTS

CONTENTS

ABOUT THE EDITORS

Anne Cawthorn, MSc, BSc (Hons), RGN, RNT, Dip Nursing, Dip Hypno, UKCP Reg, MIFPA

Anne worked as a nurse and lecturer in rehabilitation for 25 years. She moved into the field of cancer and palliative care 13 years ago, when she took up the post as Complementary Therapy Coordinator at the Neil Cliffe Cancer Centre and St Ann's Hospice. In 2000, Anne took up a joint post working as a Lecturer Practitioner with the Psycho-Oncology team at the Christie Hospital and the University of Manchester. She worked closely with her co-editor and has been involved in the integration of innovative psychological techniques and complementary therapies in the field of cancer rehabilitation. Her teaching role involved being course leader for the cancer, palliative care and com- munications-in-practice modules. Her additional areas of interest include teaching healthcare professionals to assess and manage patients' sexual and body image concerns and teaching techniques to manage anxiety and phobias. She is currently working as a Macmillan Specialist Practitioner coordinating the Living Well with Cancer Service at Blythe House Hospice in the High Peak.

Peter A. Mackereth PhD MA Dip (N) London RNT RGN

Peter is the Clinical Lead for Complementary Therapies (CTs) at The Christie NHS Foundation Trust Manchester and University Reader in Integrated Health at the University of Derby (Buxton Campus). He is a registered nurse, and has worked in intensive care, neurology and oncology. Peter has an MA in Medical Ethics and has completed a PhD project examining reflexology vs relaxation training for people with MS. In 2003, the Complementary Therapy team at the Christie received the prestigious Prince of Wales' Good Practice Award. In 2004, the team won the Department of Health's Manchester and Regional Innovations Awards in Long-term Care. In 2005, Peter was given the National Public Servant Award hosted by *The Guardian* Newspaper. The team is currently working on a number of research and audit projects exploring outcomes for acupuncture, hypnotherapy, aromatherapy, creative imagery/relaxation and reflexology. Peter has published widely and speaks regularly at conferences and study days.

CONTRIBUTORS

Ann Carter BA, Dip Health Ed, Cert Ed, MIFPA has worked in cancer care since 1993 both as a complementary therapist and co-coordinator. She works at the Christie NHS Trust as a senior therapist based in the radiotherapy and the chemotherapy suites and the relaxation 'drop ins'. Ann runs her own training consultancy and plays a major role in the development and delivery of the Integrative Therapies Training programme at the Christie. She has co-edited two books and co-authored numerous papers in professional journals.

Graeme Donald BSc DPSN RN Dip Hypno is a registered nurse and is currently working as a nurse researcher within the supportive care services at the Christie NHS Foundation Trust. He has studied hypnotherapy, medical acupuncture, creative visualization, basic massage and is committed to contributing to the development of holistic care within NHS settings. A graduate in mathematics, he integrates a scientific approach within his nursing and therapy practice and is currently undertaking a PhD researching the health benefits of Reiki for people living with HIV.

Rev. Kevin Dunn BSc, MA is Chaplaincy and Humanities Manager at the Christie NHS Foundation Trust in Manchester. After a first degree in Physics, he was a junior research assistant in the Department of Meteorology. He was ordained as an Anglican priest in 1993 and has been involved in healthcare chaplaincy since 1995. He has particular interests in literature, the arts and spirituality, and in the philosophy of healthcare.

Kevin Hinchliffe MSc, Dip Counselling, Dip Arch has practiced as an architect for the majority of his professional career. He trained as a counsellor, hypnotherapist and psychotherapist, which led to work as a Senior Therapist at the Christie and a flourishing private practice. Kevin teaches hypnotherapy, provides supervision to practitioners and has a Masters degree in Consciousness and Transpersonal Psychology.

Paula Maycock LI Biol, Hypno, LI Acu, MIFPA, MAR is a Clinical Hypnotherapist with a focus on health, wellbeing and managing stress. A Senior Therapist within the Christie NHS Foundation Trust, as well as working in private practice, Paula places emphasis on supporting patients and carers through their experiences using an integrated therapy approach. This incorporates a range of therapies and amalgamates qualifications in Clinical

Aromatherapy, Reflexology and Acupuncture with Biochemistry, Microbiology, and many years' experience working with people living with long-term illness. Paula is also proactive in promoting and supporting the use of complementary therapies and hypnotherapy in the successful attainment of a *Smoke Free* lifestyle. Paula has published and lectured within medical research and complementary medicine research fields.

Denise Rankin-Box BA (Hons) RGN Dip TD Cert ED MISMA JP initially trained in Hypnosis and Hypnotherapy in 1985. She has written and practiced hypnotherapy for over 22 years and ran a successful NHS and private Stress Management practice in the 1990s. She is Editor-in-Chief of *Complementary Therapies in Clinical Practice* and continues to write books and practice complementary medicine. Along with her husband Ian, Denise also owns Dot Medical Ltd, an innovative medical device company in the UK.

Bernadette Shepherd MSc (Integrative Psychotherapy) MSc in Nursing, BSc (Hons), RGN, Dip Nursing, CBT Cert has worked as a Registered Nurse in critical and coronary care and was a Lecturer in nursing at Manchester University. She is currently researching and developing a specialist nurse-led psychological intervention for women with breast cancer. Bernadette works part-time at the Christie NHS Trust as a psychotherapist and also runs a private psychotherapy practice for women with breast cancer who have related psychological problems. Alongside, she provides Clinical Supervision for specialist nurses at Beech Wood Cancer Care Centre.

Kathy Stephenson BA, PGCE, MSc GQHP Cert NLP, Master Practitioner is a Senior Lecturer at Sheffield Hallam University. She is the course leader of the Education, Psychology and Counselling degree course and the Certificate of Hypnotherapy. She divides her time between lecturing and running a busy private hypnotherapy/NLP practice. She has developed a range of self-hypnosis audio CDs using a combination of hypnotherapeutic suggestions, NLP techniques and creative visualization, including a CD specifically designed for children.

Julie Stone MA, LLB is an independent consultant in Healthcare Ethics and Law and visiting Professor in Ethics at the Peninsula Medical School. A lawyer by background, Julie was previously Deputy Director of the Council for Healthcare Regulatory Excellence, where she led a DH-funded project on maintaining clear sexual boundaries. She is currently a non-executive director of NHS Cornwall and the Isles of Scilly, a member of the Advisory Board on the Registration of Homeopathic Products, and senior consultant to Political Intelligence, a public affairs consultancy. A national and international expert in law, ethics and regulation of complementary and alternative medicine, she was an Advisor to the Department of Health Steering Group on the Statutory Regulation of Practitioners of Acupuncture, Herbal Medicine and Traditional Chinese Medicine, and was the author of the *Stone Report on a Federal Voluntary Structure for Regulation of CAM*.

Elizabeth Taylor M Med Sci, Dip Hyp/Psy, UKCP is a former Research Associate with a background in gastrointestinal disorders, cancer care and emotional problems. She has wide experience of psychotherapy, hypnotherapy, counselling and teaching and has published research in the field. She founded a national register of Hypno-Psychotherapists in 1993 to increase the availability of psychological support in the health service.

Lynne Tomlinson DHyp, BSCH (Assoc) 8424 is a registered clinical hypnotherapist. She works with medical and complementary therapy referrals, specializing in pain control, autoimmune disorders and anxiety states. Lynne works with the Christie Head and Neck Project dealing with emergency interventions and is a key member of a hospital-based multidisciplinary smoking cessation team, helping patients, carers and staff to go *Smoke Free*. She continues to work with smoking cessation projects both in the corporate field and in private practice. Lynne teaches Integrative Hypnotherapy, provides supervision to hypnotherapists and is currently studying for a BSc in Counselling and Complementary Medicine.

FOREWORD

Aaron Kenneth Ward-Atherton

I am both delighted and privileged to have been asked to write a foreword for this book, especially as undoubtedly, hypnotherapy will play a major role as part of a multidisciplinary approach to non-invasive therapeutics in mainstream healthcare.

Historically, Dr James Braid (1795–1860) is attributed as one of the earliest authors of hypnotism with his publication *Neurypnology* (1843). It is particularly interesting to note the analogies Braid draws between his own practice of hypnosis, and that of spirituality. The subject of spirituality in the context of hypnotherapy in itself suggests a closer relationship at a deeper emotional level, and in doing so, this publication has developed a rationale for utilizing therapeutic techniques to address those needs.

All of us at some time in our lives will be faced with realization of our own mortality; whether this be due to a disease process or simply a part of getting older, undoubtedly the experience for many will be emotionally traumatic. The strength of the book's content is it's diverse approach by skilled professionals to a wide range of illnesses and preventative measures that can be managed in an emotionally supportive way by hypnotherapy.

Cancer is no exception, and while conventional treatment is of the upmost importance, the supportive role of the complementary therapist can do much to alleviate the many cares and anxieties of the client.

I am aware that the present medical system does much to lessen suffering, but as this book illustrates, an integrative model of hypnotherapeutic intervention as an adjunctive therapy reflects the added benefits that a holistic approach can offer. No less important are the professional, legal and ethical issues surrounding the practitioner, which is intrinsically important when working with vulnerable clients, and for the protection of the practitioner in delivering good and safe practice.

The timing of this publication could not be better set against the present government directives pointing towards a patient-led health provision, with complementary therapies playing an important and integral part. To the reader, whether a healthcare professional or lay person, this work addresses the whole topic of hypnotherapy and the challenges of integrating it into present healthcare practice, by virtue of the many expert contributors.

Aaron Kenneth Ward-Atherton
Lord of Witley & Hurcott Worcestershire
Patron of the Complementary Therapies Department
The Christie NHS Foundation Trust, Manchester

FOREWORD

Bernadette Hillon

Old paint on canvass, as it ages, sometimes becomes transparent. When that happens, it is possible, in some pictures, to see the original lines: a tree will show through a woman's dress, a child makes way for a dog, a large boat is no longer on an open sea. This is called pentimento .... Perhaps it would be as well to say that the old conception, replaced by a later choice, is a way of seeing and then seeing again.

(Hellman 1976: 3)

In the Editor's introduction, Anne and Peter encourage readers to approach this book with an inquiring mind, stating they 'both believe curiosity to be an essential and empowering gift of human nature'. Few would argue that openness to inquiry and learning is also an essential hallmark of the work of practitioners and therapists. Patrick Casement (1985) wrote about this long ago, emphasizing the importance of 'learning from the patient'.

My first experience of hypnotherapeutic techniques came as a patient. Discharged from hospital following extensive abdominal surgery, my 'be strong' focus was to re-engage with life as if nothing had happened. I was soon in difficulty. No amount of thinking – my favoured approach – was helping me to dig myself out of what was becoming a larger and more complicated hole. I was somewhat bewildered but accepting of a referral to see a psychotherapist at the Neil Cliffe Centre. My journey with Anne began!

Anne worked with what I was bringing to the sessions: my dreams, imaginings, bodily sensations – the very essence of my inner experience that was hardly available for rational exploration through words. Here was someone who cared and listened and worked with my feelings, imaginings, dreams, sensations – with whatever was on and in my mind! The interventions she introduced into our work together enabled me to harness my powers of creativity, self-activation and agency at a critical time when the outlook looked bleak and my physical and emotional energies were at their lowest ebb. I was able to restore some inner sense of control in a series of life events that were largely, at that time, out of my control. Together, we co-created a space where I could explore and come to a 'new' meaning of what had happened to me, of the apprehension of what may happen in the future and of the pain and bewilderment of the present moment, as I struggled to come to terms with the impact of the surgery on my body.

I link this now to what Winnicott (1971) was discussing when he said:

... the third part of the life of a human being that we cannot ignore, is an intermediate area of experiencing, *to which inner reality and external life both contribute.*

(Winnicott 1971: 3, his emphasis on 'experiencing')

and to Jung's (1955/1956: 496) description of active imagination, 'In other words, you dream with open eyes'.

Winnicott called the 'in between' space between the conscious and the unconscious, the place where playing takes place, the 'potential space' (p. 47), 'The Place where we Live' (p. 122). Through the use of hypnotherapy I was guided into this space. I learned to 'listen' to and take notice of my inner experience – to establish a connection with myself I had not known before. I think of this now as a striving to aliveness. I realized and grasped my capacity – my 'choice' as Hellman says – to see and then see again – to reconstruct a sense of purpose in the present moment, of life going forward and a sense of my body, cut deep and scarred, coping with residual disease but alive.

I often reflect on my fortune that my therapist had the curiosity, creativity, courage and skill to offer the choice of these interventions to me as a client – interventions that were a pivotal aspect in the journey of recovery and continue to be in the maintenance of a sense of well-being in my life today.

Bernadette Hillon
Patient

BIBLIOGRAPHY

Casement, P., 1985. On Learning From the Patient. Richard Clay (The Chaucer Press), Bungay, Suffolk.

Hellman, L., 1976. Pentimento: A Book of Portraits. Quartet Books, London.

Jung, C.G., 1955/1956. Mysterium Coniunctionis. In: Read, H., Fordham, M., Adler, G., McQuire, W. (Eds.), The Collected Works of C.G. Jung, 2nd edn. vol. 14. Routledge, London.

Winnicott, D.W., 1971. Playing and Reality. Penguin Books, Harmondsworth.

ACKNOWLEDGEMENTS

The Editors would like to thank all their colleagues who contributed to this book. We appreciate that despite the personal and professional demands and challenges, they have been able to rise to the occasion and help co-create this book. It is very important that therapists, who are working in an integrative manner, have an opportunity to share their work. We hope the chapters have opened those doors and shed light on important practice developments in hypnotherapy. Special thanks go to all the patients, carers and staff, whose (anonymous) case studies have served to illuminate the integration of theory and practice within the text. We would also like to thank the Medical Illustration department (and staff who volunteered as models) at the Christie NHS Foundation Trust for their help with producing the photographs.

This book is dedicated to Diane Gray, Senior Therapist who gave 100% to her work at the Christie, the Neil Cliffe Centre/St Ann's Hospice and the Trafford Macmillan Centre. Both Anne and Peter miss her contribution to integrated care. Below is a poem written by Diane, dedicated to one of the therapists who provided support during her hospital treatment.

MY GUARDIAN ANGEL

She visits me when she can
My Guardian Angel in white
Blue eyes and bright smile
Gentle nature and care
Showing such empathy
Grace and dignity
Asking for nothing but
A belief in the Now

Her words are so unique
She has work yet to complete
Not asking how but believing
In the Now
She is so beautiful!
My Guardian Angel in white.

Written by Diane Gray

Anne Cawthorn would like to thank her colleagues and patients at the Psycho-Oncology Unit at the Christie Foundation Trust and, more recently, at The Living Well Service Blythe House. Anne would also like to give special thanks to her husband Alan for his ongoing support, and to colleagues who agreed to take on extra writing at the 'eleventh hour', namely Kathy Stephenson, Bernie Shepherd, the Reverend Kevin Dunn and Ann Carter.

Peter A. Mackereth would like to thank the staff, volunteers and patients at the Christie Foundation NHS Trust for their encouragement and inspiration. Peter would also like to acknowledge Kevin Hinchliffe and Ann Carter for being such excellent role models and teachers; Sally Olsberg for her supervision; Stephen McGinn for his support and encouragement and Keith Davies for encouraging him to keep swimming and not to take life too seriously.

Finally, a big thanks from both Anne and Peter to Linda Orrett who kindly and expertly helped with the layout and formatting of the draft manuscript.

ACKNOWLEDGEMENTS

INTRODUCTION

This book is aimed primarily at practitioners and students of hypnotherapy in the UK and internationally. Our intention is to assist in the expansion, challenge and review of existing knowledge and skills among practitioners in the best interest of patient care. The number of therapists using hypnotherapy has dramatically increased since the mid-1990s, and educational establishments are also becoming more discerning about the use of the available literature. Students attending university degree and college diploma programmes are also driving the demand for evidence-based and academic texts. Additionally, teachers also want published work that is referenced and which recommends further useful reading/resources. There are a number of key texts in hypnotherapy, and rather than supplant these, we offer with this text a practical and challenging perspective on integrated practice.

While many practitioners of hypnotherapy are health professionals, counsellors and psychotherapists, there is also an expanding workforce of bodywork therapists who have now chosen to study and utilize hypnotherapy. We believe this text creates opportunities for dialogue and debate between the various professional groups who use, teach and research hypnotherapy. Some of the ideas presented in this book will no doubt challenge some practitioners of hypnotherapy – the idea, e.g. of using touch and other complementary therapy modalities, may be a step too far for them. It could be argued that this adds complexity and makes the work harder to evaluate. Indeed, some practitioners and researchers looking for a monotherapy to solve a problem will find the content of this book choice material for criticism. It is always good to have healthy scepticism; but as optimists we are trusting that readers will engage with this book with openness and curiosity. We both agree that innovative practice needs to be tried and tested so recommend that these approaches be investigated using appropriate methodologies and outcome measures. Science begins and expands our understanding through careful observation and analysis, not by tunnel vision. The term 'placebo' is a case in point; it has come to be seen as a pejorative term, poorly understood and applied.

This book has brought together several approaches to integrating hypnotherapy. In this book there is a focus on an important area of practice – palliative and supportive care. We would like to emphasize that therapists must be able to skilfully adapt their work with individuals, and be mindful of working collaboratively with the multidisciplinary team. An important aspect of this text is that we have broadened the adaptations and value of hypnotherapy beyond the work with patients to include a 'bigger picture', so issues relating to the context in which therapeutic intervention take place are also covered.

The content of this unique book will also be of value to students, teachers and postgraduates who are looking to work safely, competently, and with compassion in the field of integrated care. There are many healthcare professionals, such as doctors, nurses, physiotherapists and occupational therapists, who have completed or want to further study hypnotherapy, so that they can expand and integrate these skills in clinical practice. This text will also be useful to coordinators of psychological, supportive complementary therapy services, as well as researchers and user/expert patient groups. The book is also intended as a resource for health professionals who provide information to patients and colleagues.

There are two sections to this book. Section 1 deals with key themes which include theoretical perspectives related to hypnotherapy, a review of the research evidence, integration issues, chapters on legal issues related to the work, PMR and the therapeutic relationship. All these themes are explored and discussed utilizing the available literature, analysis of models and concepts and are related specifically to supportive care. Section 2 focuses on innovative approaches to integrating hypnotherapy. In each of the chapters the author(s) review the available literature, propose and explore models and processes of hypnotherapy and suggest ways of adapting and incorporating other modalities. Concerns and challenges to the application of these approaches are also discussed.

This text takes the novice and the more experienced practitioner on a journey of examination, critical review and debate prior to making recommendations for best practice. Many of the ideas in this new book have evolved from the process and challenges of adapting practice in various supportive care settings, with an emphasis on using the approaches to palliative and cancer care settings within the National Health Service and the voluntary sector. There is an expectation that professional therapists will utilize contemporary information to support their practice, so that they can be reassured of person-centred, effective and, importantly, safe service. It is important to state that any recommendations made by an author(s) are to be carefully considered by the reader. They are not prescriptions to be followed without training, supervision and support. It beholds the accountable and responsible therapist to only consider an action, or inaction, in line with their codes of professional practice, where there is appropriate support of the employer/manager/supervisor and the informed consent of the client/patient. If in doubt, it is always recommended that the therapist should not proceed, and s/he should seek advice and support. It behoves the profession to become one of critical and reflective practitioners, and to acknowledge the value of research and enquiry in this process. Being and remaining curious is at the heart of the Editors' own practice, research and teaching activities. We both believe curiosity to be an essential and empowering gift of human nature. It is so easy to become complacent, and then feel and become stifled and stuck by being in a space which only permits direction and prescription. Being with others in an authentic and mindful way requires a facilitative and explorative approach to creating therapeutic relationship and best practice.

To enhance the development of professional integrated practice in supportive and cancer care, we were concerned to communicate and disseminate our understanding and appraisal of integrated hypnotherapy at this time, in order to encourage debate and appraisals of innovative practices. Indeed, we hope that the book will suggest new ideas and approaches that might be helpful to developing hypnotherapy practice in an ever-changing and complex world. This book therefore has a strong focus on adapting practice, which emphasizes key professional issues such as informed assessment of patients, reflective and supervised practice, accountability, evidence-base and health and safety issues.

Our contributors are all involved in a variety of professional activities related to hypnotherapy; including practice, research, teaching and publication. Many are also qualified health professionals, including nurses, counsellors and psychotherapists. They are respected colleagues and fellow learners in the art and science of integrated hypnotherapy. As the Editors, we would like to extend our grateful thanks to them all for their professionalism, commitment and willingness to share their expertise and experience with others.

In selecting this book for your development and studies, we feel that you are entering into a journey of exploration and discovery. We hope it will inspire you to continue learning so that you become even more creative through being curious about, and investigating ways of adapting your hypnotherapy practice. We also hope the contents of the book and your reflections upon the ideas presented support you in attaining your personal and professional potential. We are all part of a worldwide movement to acquire the necessary evidence and experience to enable true integration of hypnotherapy into a variety of healthcare settings.

Anne Cawthorn & Peter A. Mackereth

SECTION 1
KEY CONCEPTS

INTRODUCTION

This book, which explores the complementary approaches to the integrated use of hypnotherapy in clinical care, has been divided into two sections. The first part consists of six chapters, each a critical review of contemporary concepts specific to clinical practice. The authors have diverse backgrounds and training, but all have skills in teaching, supervision and therapeutic skills, with most working in supportive care settings. It is important for the reader to be aware that the book although in two parts is linked, with issues arising in Section 1 being developed in Section 2. All chapters have a short introduction and key words. Case studies are integrated within the text to illuminate both the rationale for the complementary approach and to illustrate how intervention(s) and support are tailored for the individual in clinical settings.

In Chapter 1, Denise Rankin-Box provides an introduction to the origins and history of hypnotherapy. It raises key issues relating to training and education and goes on to explore the challenges faced when integrating hypnotherapy into healthcare practice.

In Chapter 2, Kevin Hinchliffe, Anne Cawthorn, Ann Carter and Peter A. Mackereth propose an integrative model of holistic practice in which hypnotherapy techniques and other complementary approaches are offered alongside the medical model. The authors are part of a multidisciplinary team, in an acute setting, where these approaches are offered in order to enhance patient care.

In Chapter 3, Professor Julie Stone explores the professional, ethical and legal dimensions of hypnotherapy practice highlighting issues relating to consent, confidentiality. Julie discusses the need to safeguard clinical practice when working with vulnerable patients and goes on to recommend close supervision of practitioners.

In Chapter 4, Graeme Donald examines the body of evidence supporting the use of hypnotherapy in a variety of settings, offering a selection of published studies. The author discusses evidence-based practice and makes recommendations for future research projects.

In Chapter 5, Anne Cawthorn and Bernadette Shepherd review the literature surrounding the therapeutic relationship in relation to hypnotherapy. They propose the use of two models: first an assessment model and second, a model which guides hypnotherapy practice. Case studies which are based on their clinical practice as psycho-hypnotherapists in the field of cancer are included.

In Chapter 6, Peter A. Mackereth and Lynne Tomlinson present an overview of progressive muscle relaxation (PMR) development and review the research base in relation to this. The chapter offers a protocol which can form the basis in which to create PMR practice.

The development of hypnotherapy in healthcare

Denise Rankin-Box

CHAPTER CONTENTS

CHAPTER OUTLINE

The first chapter of this book describes the trance state and the origins and history of hypnotherapy. Key issues are raised with regard to training and education, private practice and the therapeutic relation. Applications within healthcare practice are briefly overviewed. The author identifies the key challenges in the greater integration of hypnotherapy in clinical practice; these will be explored in detail in subsequent chapters.

KEY WORDS

History
Trance
Stages
Education
Healthcare and application

INTRODUCTION

Hypnotherapy is often referred to as an induced state of relaxation in which the mind is more receptive to suggestion. In the main, hypnotherapy is the deliberate use of the trance state to effect change in both conscious and

© 2010 Elsevier Ltd.
DOI: 10.1016/B978-0-7020-3082-6.00003-4

unconscious states of mind. The individual and not the therapist is considered to be in control of the trance state (Rankin-Box & Williamson 2006). Although Heap and Aravind (2002) have suggested that hypnosis is an interaction between two people, it would seem that the self-induced trance state is a common daily occurrence in all people and it is not necessary for a hypnotic trance to be induced by, or dependent upon, a second party for it to occur. In this respect, self-hypnosis can be perceived as a normal state of mind.

Trance is commonly described as an altered state of consciousness. This natural state may occur several times each day (commonly referred to as day dreaming), however the neurophysiological rationale or mechanism for this is still not clearly understood. Similarly, semantic debates persist about accepted definitions of the terms hypnosis or trance. This would appear to be influenced by the way in which hypnosis and the application of the trance state is interpreted or used. Thus the social significance attributed to the function and use of the trance state can vary across cultures and sub-sects in society.

The specific induction of the trance state has formed part of many cultural practices over the centuries such as India, China, North America, Africa and Egypt (Conachy 1994). For instance, Bourguignon (1968, 1973) reported that from a sample of 488 societies, 90% had at least one socially accepted method of altering states of consciousness and trance was used in one way or another for the improvement of the individual and the community.

There are also intriguing differences in the way different social groups describe trance states. For instance, rituals involving a high degree of repetitive chanting or actions may induce trance states. Since ritual appears to be an intrinsic part of human life, it is common for people with highly ritualized lives or behaviours to be able to induce trance without specific conscious awareness until after an action has been completed, e.g. making the bed or driving to and from work when always using the same route. In such instances, trance does not block consciousness or alertness but reduces the need for the brain's neurocognitive processes to constantly monitor our actions. In contrast to this, daily existence without any ritual behaviour at all can be perceived as stressful and tiring, since a high degree of alertness is constantly required, e.g. working in a hostile environment or living with uncertainty.

Repetitive daily rituals cross all cultures and examples of highly ritualistic practice can be observed with shamanic healing, prayer, meditation, spiritual rituals, rhythmic dance, or other forms of repetitive practice. Each of these can induce the trance state.

The use of 'suggestion' in visualization, should be used cautiously to induce trance since a suggestion may not always invoke a therapeutic response, for instance, strong imagery of hot summer days in a garden full of flowers might stimulate an allergic response such as hay fever or sneezing. Suggestion, refers to the presentation of an idea to a client and the extent to which the client accepts the idea (suggestibility) is influenced by motivation and expectation. There is again, no definitive research to adequately explain this phenomenon. While suggestion remains largely psychological, it is possible using hypnotherapy, to anaesthetize parts of the body and influence the autonomic nervous system commonly considered not to be under voluntary control (Rankin-Box 2006, Whorewell et al 1992).

Anthropologically, the labels ascribed to trance induction seem to vary according to the social value placed on the significance of trance states. For some social groups, ritual trance forms a central aspect of particular ceremonies or rites of passage for its members and plays a vital part in maintaining the social cohesion of the group. It would seem that the induction of trance has been used for many centuries and across many cultures and societies. Thus the history of hypnosis should perhaps be explored in conjunction with anthropological research.

Repetitive and ritualistic actions or thoughts then, appear to predispose a state of trance. Such repetition need not occur sequentially or over a short period of time in order to invoke this state of mind. For example, individuals engaging in repetitive routines such as working on conveyor belts, or participating in rituals associated with prayer, ceremonies, healing or shamanistic practice may induce trance states. This is often remarked upon in Western society by individuals driving home from work and being unable to recall large parts of the journey home, despite having driven safely.

HISTORY

It is apparent that the origins of the use of 'trance' (more commonly termed 'hypnosis') are lost in the mists of time. Claims that the history of hypnosis originates with Franz Mesmer are misleading, since they proffer an ethnocentric approach to the use of trance within Western society and neglect the role trance has played in emergent Western civilization and other cultures.

Nevertheless, Mesmer is attributed as raising awareness of trance in Western society by the development of Mesmerism in the mid-1700s. His claim that health imbalances were affected by 'animal magnetism in the body' were perceived as revolutionary at the time and this was latterly perceived as the first medically orientated model using trance (and the use of magnets to restore magnetic balance in the body) to affect physical and psychological change. In line with other ethnographic and anthropological studies, Mesmer employed highly stylistic and theatrical rituals to induce trance his medical qualifications lent credibility and greater acceptance to his theories. However, in 1784, his work was largely discredited by the Franklin Inquiry.

Despite this, variations of Mesmer's approach to trance initiation continued to evolve. In the late 1700s, Marquis de Puysegur described a state of 'artificial somnambulism' (being asleep while awake). The Abbey de Faria referred to 'lucid sleep'. Braid referred to this as 'nervous sleep' and termed trance induction as 'Hypnotism'.

During the Second World War, Simmel developed a technique called 'hypnoanalyses for treating neurosis' (Tamin 1988). However, the word 'hypnotism' gained acceptance in Western medical circles and today hypnosis, recognized as a legitimate medical practice, continues to be acknowledged. More recently, Erikson has referred to hypnosis as 'an inner state of absorption' (Erikson & Rossi 1980). This appears as a special state described as hypnoidal or hypnotic and trance appears to be the most widely accepted term.

Erikson's approach initiated theorists of the trance 'state' and included Hilgard, Spiegel and Shatok. They argued that trance occurs after the therapist uses induction and deepening methods to guide an individual into a deep relaxation known as altered state of consciousness (ASC). Here, subjects enter a light, medium or deep trance and become responsive to suggestion as they enter deeper trance. Erickson believed that clients required an individual rather than a generic approach. However, he did believe that people already held the necessary resources to overcome their problem and hypnotic states were natural phenomena which occurred during a normal waking day. This theory currently persists and a number of these techniques form the basis of Neuro Linguistic Programming (NLP).

More recent developments in this field are described by Rankin-Box (2001, 2006), Erikson and Rossi (1980) and Spiegel and Spiegel (1978).

Although hypnosis continues to be used as a form of stage entertainment, such trance induction is induced by the individual, not the hypnotist. Thus it is not possible to induce trance against an individual's will. An individual must be willing to enter the trance state and stage hypnotists use self-induced trance to startling effect. In the UK, the Hypnotism Act of 1952 was introduced to protect the public against 'dangerous' practices when hypnosis is used for entertainment.

In 1955, the British Medical Association commenced a second inquiry into hypnosis and suggested it should be taught to psychiatrists at medical schools (British Medical Association 1955). Clinical hypnosis is now taught in medical training programmes in the USA, France and Germany. It was finally offered as a special study option for undergraduates in Medicine at the University of Oxford Medical School in 2002.

There is continuing debate as to whether hypnosis is a 'special' state or not and there is continuing debate concerning sociocognitive vs state explanations of hypnosis. State View (SV) theorists argue that there is a special state called the hypnotic trance. This state is marked by increased suggestibility, current imagery including past memories and reality distortions such as false memories. There is also a belief that future research will discover a physiological rationale for the hypnotic state. Supporters of the SV approach to hypnosis include Erickson and Spiegel. Hilgard also developed the 'Stanford Scales of Hypnotic Susceptibility, Forms A, B and C'. These scales are one of the measures currently used to objectively measure how susceptible an individual may be to hypnosis (Woody & Sadler 2005).

As early as 1960, Wyke proposed a Reality Testing Theory, also referred to as a physiological theory. Here, the process of formal hypnosis is described as involving the gradual detachment from external sensory perception (this can include closing eyes, remaining still, relaxation and focusing upon internal sensations). This form of ritualistic behaviour can create a partial suspension of reality and increases suggestibility. This could also imply a greater physiological process occurs during hypnosis than previously considered. Reducing sensory input is influenced by the reticular activating system in the central part of the brain stem and it is claimed that this may enhance patient suggestibility (Wyke 1960).

Hilgard's Neo-dissociation Theory of Hypnosis argues that individuals are constantly assessing and prioritizing events going on around us at any one time. This model suggests that the hypnotic trance modifies this arrangement so that systems become dissociated from each other and thus allowing greater critical analysis, e.g. by enhancing the ability to re-prioritize smoking from a significant daily activity and relegate it both consciously and sub-consciously to a lesser behavioural role. This argument has links with the work of Kallio and Revonsuo (2005) who suggest that the effectiveness of hypnotic analgesia might be explained as re-prioritizing perceptions of pain. Thus one can be aware of pain but develop an ability to block the neural receptors in order to reduce the sensation of pain.

The point at which an individual may be said to be 'in trance' has not yet been clearly determined. This may be due to competing theories concerning how trance is achieved and exactly what is happening during hypnosis. Future neurophysiological research may identify a physiological marker capable of defining the state constituting trance and distinguishing between the hypnotized and non-hypnotized states (Heap & Aravind 2002). However, trance appears to be a regular physiological activity of daily life. It is not neces-sarily dependent upon specific (external) trance induction. It would seem that the debate about which factors initiate trance and the extent to which this state can influence medical care and procedures will continue for some time yet.

HYPNOTHERAPY IN HEALTHCARE

Hypnotherapy is commonly associated with the induction of a trance state during which behavioural modification may be suggested. While hypnosis is a central tool, hypnotherapy tends to be a part of the interaction between the therapist and patient. The aim is to gently determine issues of concern to a patient and employ behavioural modification via hypnosis in order to bring about a beneficial and therapeutic resolution. As mentioned previously, contrary to popular belief the therapist does not take control of the client but acts only as a facilitator, helping a motivated individual towards a desired behavioural modification, e.g. smoking cessation (Rankin-Box 2006). A posi-tive desire by an individual is central to treatment success. Suggestion refers to the presentation of an idea to a client and the extent to which the client accepts the idea (suggestibility) is influenced by motivation and expectation. There is currently no definitive research to explain this phenomenon.

While suggestion remains largely psychological or a placebo-like response, it is possible to use hypnotherapy to anaesthetize parts of the body, block physiological neural transmission and affect the autonomic ner-vous system which is not usually under conscious control (Chakraverty et al 1992, Rankin-Box 2001, 2006, Whorewell et al 1992).

EXAMPLES OF APPLICATION WITHIN HEALTHCARE

Hypnotherapy has considerable potential for use within the healthcare provision and is an increasingly accepted adjunct for a range of conditions (Rankin-Box 2006). The potential applications may be broad however, as hyp-notherapy to be used effectively in the clinical setting, largely depends upon the patient's willingness to manage their own healthcare and be motivated to continue to modify their behaviour or responses to particular health problems. In this respect, the therapist is only a facilitator of the therapeutic process. Self-hypnosis may also be learnt by patients so that they are able to manage

---

BOX 1.1 Stages of hypnotherapy (Heap & Aravind 2002)

1. Induction: likened to the relaxation technique
2. Trigger: a word or action employed to induce deeper relaxation by suggestion
3. Deepening: (the ideomotor response)
4. Therapy: addressing client's concerns
5. Lightening: reorientation of the patient to their surroundings
6. Ending: reorientation of the client and the end of the trance state.

---

their own symptoms, enabling therapeutic self-sufficiency where appropriate. Given that the way in which hypnotherapy works is still being researched, it is apparent that the mind has considerable impact upon physical well-being and symptom management (see Box 1.1 for the stages of hypnotherapy). This affects both motor and autonomic responses. As a result, the extent to which hypnotherapy and self-hypnosis can create effective and beneficial health outcomes continues to be explored. However, there are currently a number of documented indications for hypnotherapy and these are listed in Box 1.2. Additionally, the overlap between hypnosis and other labels ascribed to the induction of trance states such as meditation, relaxation, shamanistic rituals, therapeutic touch, healing and so on does to some degree, mask the breadth of health benefits. To date no-one has researched the interrelationship between differing therapeutic modalities that employ repetitive or highly ritualized practices to ascertain whether these all induce the same or a similar trance state. In this respect, the therapeutic outcome could vary in direct relationship to the willingness, motivation and goal sought by the patient. Could it be that many complementary therapies attain therapeutic outcome using the same methods but under differing labels?

BOX 1.2 Potential applications of hypnotherapy with healthcare practice

- Pain management (McGlashan et al 1969)
- Control of peripheral skin temperature (Maslach et al 1972)
- Phobias (Weitzenhoffer 2000)
- Healing of burns (Edwin 1979)
- Removal of warts (Kayne 2009)
- Reducing hypertension (Benson 1977, Deabler et al 1973)
- Smoking cessation during pregnancy (Valbø & Eide 1996)
- Asthma and hyper-responsiveness (Ewer 1986)
- Wound healing and management (Rankin-Box 2006, Tamin 1988)
- Irritable bowel syndrome (Harvey et al 1989, Whorewell et al 1992, Gonsalkorale et al 2003, Al Sughayir et al 2006)
- Bronchial hyper-responsiveness in moderate asthma (Ewer & Stewart 1986)
- Insomnia (Kirsch et al 1995)
- As part of cognitive behavioural therapy (Kirsch et al 1995)
- Anxiety and anxiety associated with dentistry (Heap & Aravind 2002)
- Smoking cessation during pregnancy (Valbø & Eide 1996)
- Symptomatic management of oncology patients (nausea and pain management) (Barlow 2000).

Therapy typically lasts for 30–90 min per session and takes a number of specific stages, any one of which can be taught to the client so that they are able to practice self-hypnosis. These stages will be discussed in more depth elsewhere. Typical stages/processes used in hypnotherapy are shown in Box 1.1.

Contraindications to hypnotherapy usually involve the client's inability to maintain concentrations for long enough in order to induce or maintain trance state. Known psychological problems and borderline psychosis may also be contraindicated.

PRACTICING HYPNOTHERAPY

There are a number of issues that hypnotherapy practitioners should be aware of prior to offering therapy. Although patients may have sought out a therapist or alternatively, been referred to the therapist from another healthcare practitioner, patients have certain generic requirements for healthcare that should always be met.

AGREEING THERAPEUTIC GOALS WITH PATIENTS

Patients' perceptions of what constitutes improved care may vary from that of the provider, thus is can be helpful to clearly identify and agree patient-orientated outcome measures (Kayne 2009).

PRACTITIONER RELATIONSHIP AND GIVING INFORMATION

Pincock (2003) has noted that patients put their relationship with their doctors as second only to that of their families. Kayne (2009) suggests that this includes features as a feeling of comfort, getting support and sympathy, being told the truth and being treated as an individual. Therapists need to communicate effectively with their patients with empathy, compassion, and ensure that there is a clear understanding between therapist and patient regarding the nature of the therapy and the therapeutic outcome anticipated. Simply telling a patient about the research evidence is not enough; the evidence should be integrated with the patient's values and preferences in order to ensure individualized care occurs. Such an approach can enhance patient treatment compliance (D'Crus & Wilkinson 2005, Nolan & Badger 2005).

INVOLVING PATIENTS IN THE DECISION-MAKING PROCESS

In recent years there has been a definite move towards involving patients in the decision-making process (DMP). This is different from practitioner abdication. An example of the latter can be perceived to occur when a practitioner asks the patient 'what would you like me to do?'. Involving people in the DMP means ensuring patients are aware of the range of options available to them as well as the benefits or otherwise associated with particular choices. Thus, as Kayne (2009) notes, complementary therapy practitioners 'arrive at a course of treatment through negotiation, the patient remains in control'. In the case of hypnotherapy this is significant because trance cannot be induced nor maintained without the willingness and motivation of the patient.

PROFESSIONAL HYPNOTHERAPY PRACTICE

EDUCATION

At present, there are numerous courses available around the world. Course qualifications vary as well as course content. The length of course can also vary depending on any previous medical or allied health qualifications. There does not appear to be any standard training in hypnosis for practitioners without a medical or nursing background. At present, the British Society of Medical and Dental Hypnosis runs foundation courses and holds regular scientific meetings (Kayne 2009). However, there are a number of generic issues to consider with any course (see Box 1.3).

PRIVATE PRACTICE

In many respects, the demands placed upon hypnotherapists are similar to those of any other private or healthcare practitioner. However, due to misconceptions about the nature of trance and individual perceptions of control or lack of control while under trance, it is essential for any therapist to ensure they are well trained and have appropriate professional indemnity insurance.

Patient data and patient records are subject to legislation related to data protection and as such must be kept safe and under lock and key (see Ch. 3). Consultations should remain confidential, however on rare occasions, a therapist may become party to information that may need to be disclosed to a third party, such as medical attention or crime-related confessions that emerge during consultation. Such issues can be avoided by obtaining the client's permission to disclose specific aspects of information to a third party if expressly required in relation to instances of health and safety. This can take the form of a signed consent form between client and therapist. It should also be remembered that therapists can also choose whether to accept specific patients or not for treatment in the interests of safety or therapeutic efficacy. Thus, it may emerge during a consultation that a different therapy may be more appropriate for a client and hypnotherapy treatment stopped.

BOX 1.3 Issues to consider when choosing a course (Rankin-Box 2001, Rankin-Box & Williamson 2006)

- Is the course validated – if so by whom?
- What does the course content cover?
- Does it cover health and safety issues?
- Does the course offer a holistic approach?
- What are the qualifications of the lecturers?
- Is the course evidence-based?
- How is the course assessed?
- Does it have codes of conduct?
- Are legal and legislative issues addressed?
- Are relevant safety issues considered?

SUMMARY

Hypnotherapy has considerable potential for therapeutic efficacy within healthcare. To date it continues to be underused and undervalued. Stage acts serve to perpetuate theatrical perceptions of this therapy and undermine its value as a medical treatment. The therapeutic potential of hypnosis in facilitating autonomic conditions, has yet to be fully explored, although we do know that self-hypnosis can assist in: reducing hypertension (Kirsch et al 1995); enhancing wound healing (Tamin 1988); effectively reducing symptoms of irritable bowel syndrome (IBS) (Gonsalkorale et al 2003, Al Sughayir 2006); dental care and dental extractions; smoking and drug addiction (Valbø & Eide 1996) as well as pain management in children and during labour in childbirth (Rankin-Box 2001).

It would seem that for many people, we are not fully aware of or do not fully understand how to access the power of our own minds to stimulate healing and health responses. Perhaps the next few years will enlighten us further.

ACKNOWLEDGEMENT

Thanks go to Joanne Barber, Senior Therapist, The Christie NHS Foundation Trust, Manchester UK, for her contributions related to the theories of hypnosis.

REFERENCES

Al Sughayir, M.A., 2006. Hypnotherapy for irritable bowel syndrome in Saudi Arabian patients. East. Mediterr. Health J. 13 (2), 301–308.

Barlow, D., 2000. Unravelling the mysteries of anxiety and its disorders from the perspective of emotion theory. In: Yapko, M.D. (Ed.), Trancework and introduction to the practice of clinical hypnosis. third ed. Brunner-Routledge, New York.

Benson, H., 1977. Systemic hypertension and the relaxation response. N. Engl. J. Med. 296, 1152–1156.

Bourguignon, E., 1968. A cross cultural study of dissociated states: Final report. State University Press, Columbus.

Bourguignon, E., 1973. Religion, altered states of consciousness and social change. State University Press, Columbus.

British Medical Association, 1955. Medical uses of hypnotism. Br. J. Med. 1, Supplement: Appendix.

Chakraverty, K., Pharoah, P., Scott, D., et al., 1992. Erythromyalgia: the role of hypnotherapy. Postgrad. Med. J. 68, 44–46.

Conachy, S., 1994. Hypnotherapy. In: Wells, T.V. (Ed.), Wells' supportive therapies in healthcare. Baillière Tindall, London.

D'Crus, A., Wilkinson, J.M., 2005. Reasons for choosing and complying with complementary healthcare: an in-house study on a South Australian Clinic. J. Altern. Complement. Med. 11, 1107–1112.

Deabler, H.L., Fidel, E., Dillenkoffer, R.L., 1973. The use of relaxation and hypnosis in lowering blood pressure. Am. J. Clin. Hypn. 16 (2), 75–83.

Edwin, D.M., 1979. Hypnosis in burn therapy. In: Burrows, D.R. (Ed.), Hypnosis. Elsevier/North Holland Biomedical, Amsterdam.

Erikson, M., Rossi, E. (Eds.), 1980. In: Innovative hypnotherapy – the collected works of Milton H. Erikson on hypnosis, Vol. IV, Irvington, New York.

Ewer, T.C., Stewart, D.E., 1986. Improvement of bronchial hyper responsiveness in patients with moderate asthma after treatment with hypnotic technique: a randomised controlled trial. Br. Med. J. 293, 1129–1132.

Gonsalkorale, W.M., Mille, V., Afzal, A., 2003. Long term benefits of hypnotherapy for irritable bowel syndrome. Gut 52, 1623–1629.

Harvey, R.F., Hinton, R.A., Gunary, R.M., 1989. Individual and group hypnotherapy in treatment of refractory irritable bowel syndromes. Lancet i, 424–425.

Heap, M., Aravind, K.K., 2002. Hartlands' medical and dental hypnosis, fourth ed. Churchill Livingstone, Edinburgh.

Kallio, S., Revonsuo, A., 2005. The observer remains hidden. Contemporary Hypnosis 22 (3), 138–143.

Kayne, S.B. (Ed.), 2009. Complementary and alternative medicine. second ed. Pharmaceutical Press, London.

Kirsch, I., Montgomery, G., Sapirstein, G., 1995. Hypnosis as an adjunct to cognitive behavioural psychotherapy: a meta-analysis. J. Consult. Clin. Psychol. 63, 214–220.

Maslach, C., Marshall, G., Zimbardo, P.G., 1972. Hypnotic control of peripheral skin temperature: a case report. Psychophysiology 9, 600–605.

McGlashan, T.H., Evans, F.J., Orne, M.T., 1969. The nature of hypnotic analgesia and placebo response to experimental pain. Psychosom. Med. 31 (3), 227–245.

Nolan, P., Badger, F., 2005. Aspects of the relationship between doctors and depressed patients that enhance satisfaction with primary care. J.

Psychiatr. Ment. Health Nurs. 12 (2), 146–153.

Pincock, S., 2003. Patients put their relationship with their doctors as second only to that of their families. Br. J. Med. 327, 581.

Rankin-Box, D., 2001. Hypnosis. In: Rankin-Box, D. (Ed.), The nurses' handbook of complementary therapies. Baillière Tindall, Edinburgh.

Rankin-Box, D., Williamson, E.M., 2006. Complementary medicine: a guide for pharmacists. Churchill Livingstone, Edinburgh.

Spiegel, H., Spiegel, D., 1978. Trance and treatment: clinical uses of hypnosis. Basic Books, New York.

Tamin, J., 1988. Hypnosis. In: Rankin-Box, D. (Ed.), Complementary health therapies: a guide for nurses and the caring professions. Croom Helm, Kent.

Valbø, A., Eide, T., 1996. Smoking cessation in pregnancy: the effect of hypnosis in a randomised study. Addict. Behav. 21, 29–35.

Weitzenhoffer, A., 2000. The practice of hypnotism, second ed. Wiley, New York.

Whorewell, P.J., Houghton, L., Taylor, E., 1992. Physiological effects of emotion: assessment via hypnosis. Lancet 340, 69–72.

Woody, E.Z., Sadler, P., 2005. On the virtues of virtuosos. Contemporary Hypnosis 22 (1), 9–13.

Wyke, B.D., 1960. Neurological mechanisms in hypnosis. Some recent advances in the study of hypnosis. Royal Society of Medicine, London.

FURTHER READING

Jamieson, G. (Ed.), 2007. Toward a cognitive neuroscience of hypnosis and conscious states. Oxford University Press, Oxford.

Nash, M., Barnier, A. (Eds.), 2008. The Oxford handbook of hypnosis: theory, research, and practice. Oxford University Press, Oxford.

USEFUL RESOURCES

British Holistic Medical Association, www.bhma.org.
British Society of Clinical Hypnosis, www.bsch.org.uk.

Medical School Hypnosis Association (MSHA), www.msha.org.uk.
National Council for Hypnotherapy, www.hypnotherapists.org.uk.

The Prince of Wales Foundation for Integrated Health, www.fih.org.uk.

The Hypnotherapy Association, www.thehypnotherapyassociation.co.uk.

The General Hypnotherapy Standards Council, www.ghsc.co.uk.

The National Council of Psychotherapists, www.ncphq.co.uk.

The development of hypnotherapy in healthcare

2 An integrative model of hypnotherapy in clinical practice

Kevin Hinchliffe • Anne Cawthorn •
Ann Carter • Peter A. Mackereth

CHAPTER CONTENTS

CHAPTER OUTLINE

Our task was to consider how best to integrate hypnotherapy in clinical practice. In order to understand the relevance of the ingredients for integration we need to consider the challenges of working within healthcare settings. Included are practical issues of translating the philosophy into the practice of working with the individual in a large multidisciplinary clinical setting. In this chapter we propose a model of integrated hypnotherapy and consider the implications for education, training and research. Many of the issues raised here will be explored in further detail in subsequent chapters.

© 2010 Elsevier Ltd.
DOI: 10.1016/B978-0-7020-3082-6.00004-6

KEY WORDS

Integration
Disintegration
IHMC model
Holism
Bio-medical model

INTRODUCTION

Significant shifts in healthcare over the past 20 years have led to the development of more integrative models of healthcare in an effort to deliver patient-centred care. This has occurred alongside a demand from patients for greater information about their conventional care and a rising expectation that complementary therapies will form part of these models of care. Additionally, attitudes among the medical establishment have changed from dismissal of complementary and alternative medicine (CAM) to demands for greater regulation and evidence of safety and efficacy, in support for further integration (Molassiotis et al 2005). However, this is not the view of all medical practitioners and there is still a concerted on-going campaign against CAM, which Walach (2009) suggests might be due, in part, to the fact that CAM has grown stronger than its proponents realize.

Access to CAM varies within healthcare settings, with the greatest increase being in the field of cancer and palliative care. Corner and Harewood (2004) support this view, suggesting that the use of CAM in this group may be higher than in the general population. When reviewing the literature, a variety of reasons are given for the increasing use of CAM among patients who have cancer. Their use can be placed on a continuum. At one end, their use is a purely pleasurable intervention, while at the other end, they have an enhancing affect on the patient's quality of life. Their role may be to complement or counteract the side effects of conventional cancer treatments. Cassileth (1998) suggests that CAM has a variety of uses which range from support for patients' psychological needs, to dissatisfaction with the medical system and/or as a result of a poor relationship with their physicians.

While acknowledging that the use of CAM in healthcare settings, and by the general population, is a way of helping individuals to manage their own self-care and symptom control, it is important to develop models of care which ensure that therapies are safe, appropriate and aim to avoid harm. Tavares (2006) suggests that there are three main elements that need to be considered when integrating complementary therapies into supportive and palliative care and these are: accountability, evidence-based care and the multidisciplinary approach.

ACCOUNTABILITY

Over the past 12 years, government strategies which aim to ensure that quality of care becomes the driving force for the development of health services in England have been central to many reports (DoH 1997, 1998, 2008, NICE 2004). Clinical governance frameworks also provide health service organizations with clear directives on what constitutes commitment to quality and the safeguarding of standards (DoH 1999). However, Peters (2009) suggests that the government is now seeking ways of delivering compassion in the NHS. This follows on from the NHS Review (DoH 2008: 11) in which Lord Darzi states that the NHS 'provides round the clock, compassionate care and comfort ... [that] ... should be as safe and effective as possible, with patients treated with compassion, dignity and respect'.

EVIDENCE-BASED PRACTICE

Evidence-based care has been described by Sackett (1996) as the conscientious, judicious and explicit use of current best evidence when making decisions about the care of individual patients. The need for evidence-based integrative medicine is one of great concern (Dooley 2009). Stone (2002) believes that because of the absence of a credible research base within CAM it has been used as a political stick to hamper attempts at integration. Hypnotherapy practitioners need to integrate the best available evidence into their clinical practice so as to ensure safety and efficacy while ensuring they also do no harm (see Ch. 4).

MULTIDISCIPLINARY APPROACH

Integrated care involves a patient-centred holistic approach, which aims to meet the needs of each individual patient. This approach involves all health professionals and therapists working together, in partnership with patients, to maximize their potential for health and well-being. Tavares (2006) suggests that the delivery of integrated care demands a willingness to collaborate, from both conventional and complementary therapy professionals. Whether hypnotherapy is being offered within healthcare or in a private setting, the therapist should link with the patient's multidisciplinary team by communicating his/her role in supporting the patient and expected outcomes, as a contribution to the patient's overall care.

One way of ensuring that collaboration is undertaken is through the utilization of a model, in which there is mutual understanding of what integrated care entails.

In the past, these interventions may have been offered by a range of separate healthcare professionals, or indeed, interventions such as hypnotherapy were not offered at all. Dixon (2009) comments that what is emerging in general practice is akin to Lord Darzi's polyclinic plan. The plan suggests that the future GP will offer a much more integrative approach. This will include a whole person approach, for the GP to be an expert in helping patients to help themselves to improve personal health, and to be able to discuss the widest range of safe and effective treatment options, which may include CAM. He further adds that the GPs could have some skills in CAM offering them as part of their work. This view, already practiced by some, would fit in with the integrative model of holistic care (IMHC), which is discussed below.

However, the concept of 'integrated medicine' has been criticized by Ernst (2009). He suggests that it is a superfluous term which implies that conventional medicine ignores holistic care. Integrated care is argued to be a 'whole' person approach (Dixon 2009) which extends beyond the biomedical model of disease to encompass health and well-being (Rees & Weil 2001). It is a positive approach that considers the causes (e.g. smoking, obesity and lack of exercise) *and* causes at a personal, social and spiritual level (e.g. stress, low self-esteem and negative messages). Medical care has been criticized as having become so industrialized that it has narrowed its vision to 'fixing' the human machine and then treating the side-effects of the technology, rather than being interested in health and healing (Barraclough 2007, WHO 1998). Some patients expect to receive the 'magic bullet' which perpetuates the 'cure me, but don't ask me to consider changing my lifestyle'. The integrated approach must start before conception and in early childhood to empower communities, families and individuals to engage and take charge of their own health and well-being. For example, in smoking cessation, hypnotherapy cannot stop someone from smoking. However, it can open the door to explore an understanding of why the person smokes and what resources can help them change (see Ch. 10). It is also about working with families, friends, in the wider community and in the workplace.

THE INTEGRATIVE MODEL OF HOLISTIC CARE

In order to support patients, hypnotherapists need to have a way of working which helps them to provide safe holistic care. This can include working with an integrative model that is complementary to the patient's medical care (Cawthorn 2006). The integrative model of holistic care (IMHC) attempts to do this (Fig. 2.1). The model draws on work undertaken in the field of oncology and palliative care by Kearney (1997, 2000) and has been adapted by Cawthorn and Mackereth (2005), Cawthorn (2006) and Molassiotis et al (2005) in an

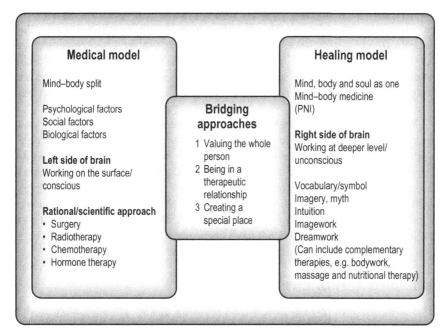

FIG 2.1 The integrative model of holistic care (IMHC).

attempt to conceptualize how CAM can be better integrated in different areas of healthcare practice. This approach to care aims to work with the whole person, mind, body and soul, in supporting them through the unique response to their illness. It involves using mind–body medicine, alongside their medical programme, to facilitate personal growth and self-healing.

The IHMC has the following three aspects:

THE HEALING MODEL

The healing aspect of the model is represented on the right hand side of Figure 2.1. Working in this domain lends itself to the use of hypnotherapy as the therapist works with the unconscious, using intuition, symbol, imagery and myth, which can include the use of imagework and dreamwork (Kearney 2000). It also links in with the state of trance which CAM practitioners can access as part of the therapeutic approach. Working in this way links in with research from the emerging field of psychoneuroimmunology (PNI). There is now a substantial amount of evidence into the mind (psychology), the brain (neurology) and the body's natural defences (immunology), to suggest that the mind and body communicate with each other (Ader 1996) (see Ch. 6). This has been made possible through a rapid advance in the scientific understanding of the immune system over the past 30 years. The concept that every thought, idea and belief is part of the mind–body pathways raises interesting questions into the role of these in maintaining health and fighting disease.

THE MEDICAL MODEL

This is illustrated on the left hand side of Figure 2.1. Kearney (2000) contrasts the approach of the medical model, where the emphasis is placed on the conscious mind. Cunningham (2000) reminds us that the medical model with its mind–body split and care, often ignores the more emotional and existential aspects relating to a diagnosis of cancer or any other life-threatening or life-limiting illness. Medicine has been criticized for its paternalism, which, while well meaning, can be experienced as disempowering, preventing an individual taking responsibility and ownership of their bodies, lives, families and communities (Illich 1979).

The adoption of an integrative model has benefits for both patients and practitioners and many doctors are now looking to offer an integrated approach which recognizes the whole person, not just their medical needs (Dixon 2009). This requires greater communication from all practitioners involved in the patient's care. A hypnotherapist needs to have an awareness of the diagnosis and treatments which a patient may be undertaking, even though they may not be directly involved with these. Communication can be in many forms, from letters, accessing patient's notes, being involved in ward rounds, or through adoption of patient-held records.

BRIDGING APPROACHES

The bridging approaches are a way of working and ideally should form the philosophy from which all the practitioners involved in integrative health should work. In essence, it is what binds the two areas of work together and the compassion, respect and dignity shown by all the team members should be evident to the patients within their care. There are three core components:

1. Valuing the whole person
2. Being in a therapeutic relationship
3. Creating a 'Special Space' for the work.

Valuing the whole person

Through the adoption of the IMHC model the hypnotherapist works with and values every aspect of the patient. Working with the conscious and unconscious aspects of the patient involves respecting what emerges as part of the therapy. Bollentino (2001: 101) suggests that 'each person is an organic whole, with inseparable physical, intellectual, psychological, social, creative, and spiritual aspects'. Most people do not routinely tune into all these aspects of themselves and hypnotherapy can facilitate this process. This may entail the therapist helping the patient to adjust to the changes which occur as a result of the patient's individual and unique response to their illness and subsequent treatments.

Being in a therapeutic relationship

The second core component is the therapeutic relationship, which is essential for all therapeutic encounters. The importance of developing the therapeutic relationship is recognized within both the field of healthcare and CAM. Erskine et al (1999) see the relationship as the key component, recommending that it should be nurtured and entered into fully, as it is a vehicle for growth and healing. For practitioners to sustain effective therapeutic relationships, reflective practice, clinical supervision and being open to the journey of personal growth and development are recommended (Mackereth 1997). Developing an affirmation statement, such as the one below, may be useful for staying focused and present in therapeutic relationships:

> [to have] ... an open heart, a willingness to journey with others, but acknowledge that I have my own needs and issues for which I require support. I believe healing can take place if I can be with others and be myself in a way that defines our boundaries and helps to create sacred space for shared healing.
>
> (Mackereth 1998: 127)

The therapeutic relationship is discussed in depth and is further developed in Chapter 5.

Creating a 'Special Space'

The third aspect at the core of this model is the creation of a 'Special Space'. This 'space' is about creating a holding environment where one person can attune to the other's needs.

It is important to note that when faced with illness and disability, patients can experience an emergence of hidden or even repressed emotion when their bodies receive nurturing and support in a safe and therapeutic space. Crucially from a healing perspective, these responses can be powerfully cathartic, especially when witnessed and acknowledged by another, whose compassion and willingness to be present is clearly evident. The 'Special Space' between the therapist and patient, is where the potential for healing the soul can occur. It is akin to Bion's (1962) definition of containment, which involves 'being there' with others in their suffering. This includes an ability to contain their emotional material as the patients will only feel secure if they know that the therapist can contain their suffering and not be overwhelmed by it. However, this does not always mean being able to make it better, but it does involve the capacity to create a holding environment.

Working in this way requires the therapist to have undergone sufficient training, be receiving supervision and be part of, or linked to, a team to whom this work is familiar. One way of ensuring this, is for the hypnotherapy practitioner to bring the 'three Ps' into his/her therapeutic work. These are Potency, Protection and Permission (Crossman 1966) and have been used as a framework to explore practice issues in clinical supervision (Mackereth 1997). First, the patient needs to know and feel that their practitioner is 'potent' in their work, to feel confident and trusting of their skills. Potency, for the practitioner, is having and acknowledging specialized skills developed and sustained by being open to learning (Stewart 1989). This is especially important when using hypnotherapy. Potency means being clear about the contract for the work; this can help to develop 'protection' for both patient and practitioner (Stewart 1989).

BOX 2.1 Some challenges and strategies for greater integration

Practice	Research	Education and training
▪ Multidisciplinary meeting – opportunities for complementary therapists to contribute	▪ Mixed methods – beyond the RCT	▪ Shared learning opportunities – conferences/study days
▪ HCPs need to observe hypnotherapy in practice	▪ Importance of reporting patient narratives	▪ Educate HCPs about hypnotherapy theory
▪ Therapists require exposure to medical practice/diagnostic/ interventions	▪ Explorative forms of enquiry	▪ Opportunities for HCPs to experience hypnotherapy
▪ HCPs to recognize the impact of language on stress and anxiety	▪ Researchers need to bring therapists on board rather than alienate	▪ To sign post services of regulated and suitable trained therapists
▪ Develop criteria for the 'when' and 'why' to refer for hypnotherapy	▪ Therapists skilled in hypnotherapy should be advisors on studies	
	▪ Current and skilled practice needs to be evaluated	
	▪ Need to capture practice not reduce it – account for variables not eliminate them	
	▪ Need for greater equity in funding	
	▪ Academia needs to show interest in hypnotherapy research development	

HCPs, Healthcare professionals; this includes students.

Permission is also very important and is a two-way process. The hypnotherapy practitioner needs to give the patient permission to share their concerns, and this may include any images and dreams which emerge as part of embarking on this work. The patient also needs to understand and consent to hypnotherapy techniques before the therapist begins using trancework.

INTEGRATION OF HYPNOTHERAPY IN PRACTICE

An integrated model of hypnotherapy applicable to a variety of healthcare settings should by definition be all-inclusive. The reality is perhaps more elusive, given the complexity of care and the support needed both practically and financially to provide hypnotherapy in clinical settings. It may feel more like a happy coincidence when a service is able to resource knowledgeable and competent therapists who are able to offer hypnotherapy at the right time and with the right patients. No one individual can be the right therapist in all possible healthcare situations. While the model proposed in this chapter represents a philosophical approach rather than a step-by-step guide, there are three key elements to the practice of hypnotherapy.

Medical and dental practitioners who understand the procedures and theories underlying the application of hypnosis could also incorporate the practice, where applicable, into their work. Doctors and other health professionals do not need to be the only ones to learn and practice hypnosis. Indeed, we argue that suitably trained practitioners can be employed to help widen access to this intervention. To become more fully integrated, it is our belief that hypnotherapy needs to step beyond its current 'adjunct' status within medical and dental practice.

Many complementary therapies have, in common with hypnotherapy, the induction of states of relaxation (see Ch. 8). An understanding of hypnotherapeutic techniques would be of enormous value to complementary therapists who may unintentionally trigger trance states during treatments. Do we tell patients that during many therapies they can access a deeper relaxation of mind as well as body? If we remove or alleviate temporarily the feelings of anxiety, stress or worry, inner resources become more accessible. It is possible that when profoundly relaxed, problems which seemed insurmountable can become curious puzzles to be solved.

First, the therapist can offer 'imagery': this term is used in preference to the term 'visualization' (see Ch. 8). Using the 'imagination' can include visual, auditory, kinaesthetic, olfactory and gustatory senses. The ability to create metaphorical images in relation to physiological or psychological conditions can be a powerful way of making the changes necessary in gaining some influence and control over the offending condition. For example, when we drift off while driving or walking, we normally utilize one or more of these senses to create or remember the world within our mind. This 'chatter' has purpose; it enables us to ponder and gain understanding or insight. Sometimes the thinking gets stuck. This can lead us to seeking help or we may remain in an anxious state if we do not believe that the inner resources needed to resolve a situation are available to us. Hypnotherapy can help to manage the 'chatter' or redirect it profitably, depending on the person's needs. For example, for healthcare professionals, the integration of this process in clinical practice is relevant to preventing and minimizing needle anxiety – where fear preoccupies the individual and interferes with the ability to tolerate cannulation (see CALM, Ch. 7 for examples).

Second, the power of 'suggestion' can be effective in introducing ideas or questions, which might imply a solution to a problem. A suggestion made can be absorbed by the subconscious mind if it is considered beneficial to the patient. The therapist has to be skilled and responsible in the use of the art of suggestion. In practice, this can help to clarify the difference between stage hypnotism and clinical use of hypnotherapy. Suggestions which are made to an individual to behave in a certain way can be achieved on stage; the person in this context has consented to be part of an entertainment. However, in clinical work, a patient will not accept a suggestion to 'stop smoking', unless s/he has the motivation, knowledge and resources to modify smoking behaviours.

Finally, hypnotherapy can be used to explore the subconscious mind, to bypass (with permission) the critical censor of the conscious mind, allowing the interface between the conscious and unconscious, which results in the client having the information they need to make any necessary changes (American Society for Clinical Hypnosis 2009). It can be safely used to uncover experiences, which may be blocking progress and identify resources, which the client may have to assist in the consciously expressed desire for improved well-being. At the practical level, for any integration to happen, all boundaries should be flexible. Where the primary discipline is medical care, then hypnotherapy should be considered as a complement to that process, enabling the process to be more effective.

BEING AN INTEGRATED MEMBER OF THE MULTIDISCIPLINARY TEAM

This requires the therapist to adhere to policies and standard operating procedures within the organization. The therapist must be prepared to complete records of all interventions. This is not only good practice from a therapy stance; it is essential from a legal position and would normally be a management requirement. Access to patients for therapy sessions within healthcare may be in very different environments to those afforded in private practice. The therapist needs to be able to work in curtained cubicles, noisy wards, or in therapy rooms where external noises are impossible to control. Also interruptions can occur and it is always important to build in the potential for any noise into the initial discussion and as part of the therapy script. For example, 'with every sound that you hear you will become more and more relaxed.' It is important to remember that the therapist needs to be calm and grounded, to have set up a 'sacred space' between themselves and the patient, and have sufficiently developed the relationship so that they are a companion on the journey. In such a relationship, extraneous noises often pale into insignificance (see Case study 2 in Ch. 5). Case study 1 in Box 2.2 demonstrates how hypnotherapy forms part of multiprofessional working.

BOX 2.2 Case study 1

Rosanna, aged 26, was anxious about a medical investigation which required hospital admission. She revealed that she had a panic attack the last time that this procedure was performed and was anxious to avoid this happening again. She also revealed that she had suffered from depression in the past and feared that this may be starting again as she was aware that her mood was dropping. During the weekly triage meeting, it was decided who would be the best person to support Rosanna. As the therapist was not trained as a mental health worker, it was decided that she would be offered an assessment and ongoing support from the psychologist. It was also agreed that the therapist would share care for Rosanna during the week she was hospitalized. Creative Imagery and Progressive Muscle Relaxation training (see Ch. 6) was provided to help relieve Rosanna's anxiety. The psychologist helped Rosanna to explore her concerns and reinforced the value of the interventions offered. No medication was required.

IDENTIFYING THE BOUNDARIES OF PRACTICE

It is essential that the therapist works within the boundaries of his/her competence within the context of the responsibilities of the wider care team. The practitioner may be a healthcare professional, e.g. doctor, dentist, psychiatrist, nurse, counsellor, psychotherapist, psychologist or complementary therapist. Psychiatrists, psychologists and mental health nurses will normally assess, refer and offer/prescribe interventions for people living with mental health conditions. Therapists using hypnotherapy, without these trainings, may come into contact with patients experiencing mental health problems, which are not formally diagnosed. Opportunities must exist in healthcare settings to triage or sort roles and responsibilities with regard to the best interest of the patient.

EDUCATION AND TRAINING

Shared learning opportunities provide time with other professionals to understand each others' contribution, professional views and concerns. It also helps to clarify boundaries and consider future shared working. Polarization of views will continue without multiprofessional appreciation of roles. Expert patient programmes and access to information via the internet, the latter not always of good quality, are levellers with informed users of services equipped to question healthcare professionals and be fully informed prior to procedures, treatments and care. Comprehensive care packages need to acknowledge that the patient has already made choices, irrespective of the views of healthcare staff. For example, it is common for patients not to share with medical and nursing staff that they are also pursuing complementary and alternative therapies, including hypnotherapy, for fear of being judged.

The therapist needs to become an interactive member of the team rather than an isolated practitioner with expertise which is not on show or shared (see Boxes 2.1 and 2.3). There are aspects of physiology, psychology and spirituality involved in the total model and it would be brave to suggest that an

> **BOX 2.3 Case study 2**
>
> Having observed therapists using hypnotherapy within a chemotherapy day unit, a senior member of the nursing staff requested some tips on relaxation skills to help continue the work of a therapist. She suggested staff could observe the hypnotherapist in action and then practice with subsequent patients. Having considered the request, it was suggested that observation was a good idea, with the patient's permission, but suggested that a short course over three afternoons be arranged to include teaching relaxation techniques (not hypnotherapy), theory and practice away from the chemotherapy day unit. Included was a session of use of language to facilitate a calm and positive approach to cannulation (see case studies in Ch. 7).

individual practitioner could be expert in all aspects. Opportunities exist or can be provided through continuing professional development (CPD) events for all healthcare professionals to gain understanding of the power of the patient's subconscious ability to become an active ingredient in the treatment. Indeed, it would be helpful to have knowledge of and exposure to clinical hypnotherapy practice before making a judgement (see Box 2.1).

INTEGRATED APPROACH TO RESEARCH

Evidence-based medicine to treat medical conditions is to be applauded and double-blinded randomized controlled trials have their place. Evidence-based interventions to support individuals to manage their health and well-being demands more complex forms of investigations, which includes listening to the individual's narrative. Science has found truly awe-inspiring treatments for diseases such as TB and ways of intervening in HIV progression to AIDS. Yet those diseases continue to spread and become resistant to medication. Prevention of disease and compliance to treatment go beyond the scope of a randomized controlled trial. Research methodologies must be adaptable and able to take account of the complex world in which many individuals, families and communities of the world struggle to maintain an existence. With clinical hypnotherapy practice, where no two patients are alike and where the therapy itself is a journey with choices and where helpful strategies emerge rather than being dictated by the therapist. The patients and their resources are the treatment rather than a medicine or technique. Research has its place in evaluating safety, efficacy and effectiveness of hypnotherapy; the danger is the tunnel vision of some of its practitioners. It is essential not to stifle curiosity by imposing one view of research. Research funding is essential yet very little is available for evaluating CAM. Hypnotherapy, in terms of its nuances of practice occupies the same complexity of territory as psychotherapy and counselling. Indeed physiotherapy, occupational therapy and nursing are practiced using a variety of technical, interpersonal and facilitator skills. Box 2.4 describes a scenario where hypnotherapy expertise is required in reviewing a research proposal. A review of the research evidence and key issues related to methodology are presented in Chapter 4.

BOX 2.4 Scenario I

A researcher has approached a hypnotherapy team to assist in a research project. His plan is a randomized controlled trial comparing hypnotherapy with a standard care arm. Both arms of the trial would receive the usual postoperative medication, with one group also receiving hypnotherapy. The aim of the pilot project would be to investigate if hypnotherapy reduced the use of pain medication (all participants would be given a patient-controlled analgesic syringe driver). The researcher proposed that the senior hypnotherapist would teach nurses to hypnotize patients postoperatively daily for 5 days using a standard protocol or script each time for 20 minutes.

The team discussed this proposal and suggested that a project might be possible, but the sessions would need to be individualized and provided preoperatively by the hypnotherapy team. The nurses' role would be to encourage patients to practice the instilled technique and contact the hypnotherapy team for support, if needed. The study would of course need ethical and access approval.

CONCLUSION

An integrative approach to clinical hypnosis needs to recognize the art as well as the science; the subconscious as well as the conscious. Appreciating the patient's own voice, experiences, values and beliefs (spiritual) are integral to meeting the person within the therapeutic work. The therapists therefore must value the process as well as the procedures. The therapist needs to recognize and understand that the key to the work lies primarily in facilitation of the client's own access to resources (direction not instruction).

In working as part of a wider health service, a model of practice has been proposed. Within this model a bridge between the two paradigms (e.g. health and disease – facilitation and prescriptions) needs to be secured. The process of greater integration of hypnotherapy in practice does identify important challenges; these have been identified here and will be explored in more detail elsewhere in the book. As the Prince of Wales has suggested, we should be seeking and valuing the best of both complementary and conventional medicine in the best interest of the health and well-being of patients (Prince Charles HRH 2001).

REFERENCES

Ader, R., 1996. Historical perspectives on psychoneuroimmunology. In: Friedman, T.W., Klein, T.W., Friedman, A.L. (Eds.), Psychoneuroimmunology, stress and infection. CRTC Press, Boca Raton.

American Society for Clinical Hypnosis, 2009. Information for the general public. Online Available: http://asch.net/genpublicinfo.htm.

Barraclough, J., 2007. Introducing the holistic approach to cancer care. In: Barraclough, J. (Ed.), Enhancing cancer care: complementary therapy and support. Oxford University Press, Oxford.

Bion, W.R., 1962. The psycho-analytic study of thinking. A theory of thinking. Int. J. Psychoanal. 43, 306–310.

2

KEY CONCEPTS

Bollentino, R.C., 2001. A model of spirituality for psychotherapy and other fields of mind-body medicine. Adv. Mind Body Med. 17, 90–107.

Cassileth, B.R., 1998. The alternative medicine handbook: the complete guide to alternative medicine. Norton, New York.

Cawthorn, A., 2006. Working with the denied body. In: Mackereth, P., Carter, A. (Eds.), Massage and bodywork adapting therapies for cancer care. Churchill Livingstone, Edinburgh.

Cawthorn, A., Mackereth, P., 2005. Complementary and alternative therapies in rheumatology. In: Hill, J. (Ed.), Rheumatology nursing. second ed. Whurr, London.

Corner, J., Harewood, J., 2004. Exploring the use of complementary and alternative medicine by people with cancer. J. Nurs. Res. 9 (2), 101–109.

Crossman, P., 1966. Permission and protection. Transactional Analysis Bulletin 5 (19), 152–154.

Cunningham, A.J., 2000. The healing journey: overcoming the crisis of cancer. Key Porter Books, Toronto.

Dixon, M., 2009. General practice – the future is integrated. Journal of Holistic Healthcare 6 (1), 5–6.

Dooley, M., 2009. An integrated approach to gynaecology. Journal of Holistic Healthcare 6 (1), 44–47.

DoH, 1997. The new NHS: modern, dependable. CM 3807. The Stationery Office, London.

DoH, 1998. A first class service: quality in the new NHS. The Stationery Office, London.

DoH, 1999. Clinical governance: quality in the new NHS. NHS executive, Department of Health, Leeds.

DoH, 2008. High quality care for all: NHS next stage review final report. Dept of Health, London. Online Available: www. dh.gov.uk/en/Publicationsandstatistics/ PublicationsPolicyAndGuidance/ DH085825.

Ernst, E., 2009. Integrated medicine: the best of both worlds and the worst for our patients? Complement. Ther. Med. 17 (3), 179–180.

Erskine, R.G., Moursund, P., Trautmann, R. J., 1999. Beyond empathy: a therapy of contact-in relationship. Edwards Brothers, Michigan.

Illich, I., 1979. Limits to medicine. Marion Boyars, London.

Kearney, M., 1997. Mortally wounded: stories of soul pain, death and healing. Touchstone, New York.

Kearney, M., 2000. A place of healing: working with suffering in living and dying. Oxford University Press, Oxford.

Mackereth, P.A., 1997. Clinical supervision for 'potent' practice. Complement. Ther. Nurs. Midwifery 3, 38–41.

Mackereth, P., 1998. Body, relationship and sacred space. Complement. Ther. Nurs. Midwifery 4 (5), 125–127.

Molassiotis, A., Cawthorn, A., Mackereth, P., 2005. Complementary and alternative therapies in cancer care. In: Kearney, A., Richardson, A. (Eds.), Nursing patients with cancer. Elsevier Science, London.

NICE, 2004. Guidance on Cancer Services. Improving supportive and palliative care for adults with cancer. National Institute for Clinical Excellence, London.

Peters, D., 2009. Integration, long term disease and creating a sustainable NHS. Journal of Holistic Healthcare 6 (1), 29–31.

Prince Charles, H.R.H., 2001. The best of both worlds. Br. Med. J. 322, 181.

Rees, L., Weil, A., 2001. Integrated medicine imbues orthodox medicine with the values of complementary medicine. Br. Med. J. 322, 119–120.

Sackett, D.L., Rosenberg, W.M., Gray, J.A., et al., 1996. Evidence based medicine: what it is and what it isn't. Br. Med. J. 312 (7023), 71–72.

Stewart, I., 1989. Transactional analysis counselling in action. Sage, London.

Stone, J., 2002. An ethical framework for complementary and alternative therapists. Routledge, London.

Tavares, M., 2006. Integrative practice. In: Mackereth, A., Carter, A. (Eds.), Massage & Bodywork: adapting therapies in cancer care. Elsevier Science, London.

Walach, H., 2009. The campaign against CAM – a reason to be proud. Journal of Holistic Healthcare 6 (1), 8–13.

WHO, 1998. WHOQOL and spirituality, religiousness and personal beliefs Report on WHO Consultation. WHO, Geneva.

FURTHER READING

Barraclough, J. (Ed.), 2007. Enhancing cancer care: complementary therapy and support. Oxford University Press, Oxford.

Heller, T., Lee-Treweek, G., Katz, J., et al., 2005. Perspectives on complementary and alternative medicine. Routledge, Taylor & Francis, Abingdon.

USEFUL RESOURCES

British Holistic Medical Association, PO Box 371, Bridgwater, Somerset TA6 9BG. Tel: 01278 722 000; e-mail: admin@bhma.org; website: www.bhma.org.uk.

The Prince's Foundation for Integrated Health, PO Box 65104, London SW1P 9PJ. Tel: 020 7024 5755; e-mail: contactus@fih.org.uk; website: www.fih.org.uk.

An integrative model of hypnotherapy in clinical practice

3

Professional, ethical and legal issues in hypnotherapy

Julie Stone

CHAPTER OUTLINE

This chapter will explore some of the professional, ethical and legal dimensions of hypnotherapy practice, including: a review of its current regulatory status and safeguards in maintaining professional practice. The author also explores issues related to consent, confidentiality, working with vulnerable patients and the importance of supervision and relation of practitioners.

© 2010 Elsevier Ltd.
DOI: 10.1016/B978-0-7020-3082-6.00005-8

Law
Ethics
Professional practice
Risk
Confidentiality
Autonomy

INTRODUCTION

Hypnotherapy is increasingly recognized as a standalone therapy, or as a useful adjunct to other conventional and integrated therapeutic modalities. Like all forms of therapy, hypnotherapy has the capacity to bring about benefits, but also the capacity to cause harm. Most risks in practice are predictable, and are minimized if hypnotherapy is provided by suitably trained, regulated practitioners in safe practice settings.

A practitioner's responsibilities fall into three broad areas relating to: respecting autonomy, benefiting patients and not harming them, and demonstrating respect for principles of justice. Specific issues explored will include consent, confidentiality and its limits, working within limits of competence, avoidance of harm, working as part of a multidisciplinary team, and safety and clinical governance issues.

Public misperceptions around hypnotherapy arise, in no small part, because of the association with stage hypnosis, and the inducing of trance for the purpose of entertainment. The confusion between hypnosis and hypnotherapy gives rise to concern that hypnotherapists are able to make people submit to their will while 'under their spell'. This perception is not representative of hypnotherapy used as a therapeutic technique, which the UK House of Lords' Science and Technology Select Committee defined as: 'the use of hypnosis in treating behavioural disease and dysfunction, principally mental disorders.' In this context, hypnotherapy is employed solely for the benefit of patients. Nonetheless, the fears conjured by lack of understanding about the remit of hypnotherapy need to be addressed, because they go to the heart of issues of control, power in the therapeutic relationship, best interests and therapeutic intent. As with all therapeutic endeavours, the focus of treatment should be in the best interests of the patient. Patients themselves must decide whether they wish to undergo, receive or participate in any given therapy, and the giving of information is a key responsibility of practitioners, reflected in the law through the duty to obtain consent.

WHY ETHICS AND LAW ARE AN ESSENTIAL PART OF PROFESSIONAL PRACTICE

Healthcare relationships are based on trust. Patients rely on practitioners to act in their interests at all times. The power imbalance inherent in all healthcare professional relationships requires hypnotherapists to be sensitive to the ethical implications of the therapeutic encounter. Patients are often, but not always, anxious or vulnerable, and assume that therapists know what they are doing, and working within the scope of their competence. The patient's beliefs are shaped by the environment in which treatment is offered, the white coat (if worn), and the use of technical language, which frame the professional encounter. Professionalism implies 'service to others'. This reflects the fiduciary nature of the relationship between any therapist and patient. The offer to heal is extremely potent, and it is vital that hypnotherapists do not abuse their patient's trust, overstate their own capabilities, or make unrealistic claims about what treatment can offer. Critically, the foundation of the professional relationship is based on the *best interests of the patient*, and not the convenience or financial advantage of the practitioner.

There are obvious reasons why practitioners should work within the law. The main reason is that healthcare laws, relating e.g. to consent and confidentiality, are in place to protect the rights of the patient. Additionally, working within the law, including keeping good records of what has been said and done, acts as a protection for practitioners in the event of any dispute arising out of treatment, which may result in a complaint to employers or a professional disciplinary tribunal. The key ethical and legal issues for hypnotherapists are set out in Box 3.1.

BENEFITING AND NOT HARMING

The main ethical issue in any given modality is the need to benefit patients and not cause harm. This reflects the key principles of beneficence and non-maleficence, cornerstones of professional ethics. For any treatment to be offered, its benefits should outweigh its risks, and treatment should, so far as is possible, be evidence-based. Benefits of hypnotherapy may be specific (e.g. a reduction in symptoms) or broader (e.g. an enhanced sense of well-being or optimism). Arguments exist around *who* should determine what constitutes a benefit, and conventional medicine has tended to look for measurable benefits to provide some objective, verifiable evidence as to

---

BOX 3.1 Key ethical and legal issues

- Working within the limits of competence
- Keeping good records
- Being aware of the contraindications to hypnotherapy, including working with vulnerable groups
- Undertaking continuing professional development (CPD) and receiving appropriate supervision
- Empowering patients by ensuring they fully understand and consent to hypnotherapy
- Maintaining confidentiality
- Creating and maintaining effective professional boundaries
- Responding appropriately and effectively to complaints
- Acting on concerns about other practitioners.

effect. Risks may also be specific, e.g. exacerbation of symptoms (or causing side-effects) and non-specific, e.g. loss of confidence in health professionals, and contributing to patients not seeking other forms of treatment from which they might benefit.

RISKS AND BENEFITS OF HYPNOTHERAPY

As stated, the risks and benefits relate both to therapies and individual practitioners, and each needs to be considered separately. As regards the therapy itself, patients may not be aware of what the purported benefits of hypnotherapy are, so practitioners who use hypnotherapy, either on its own, or as part of other treatment pathways, should be in a position to articulate what the anticipated benefits of this therapy are. Information leaflets can be a helpful way of setting out the main benefits of treatment and any anticipated side-effects. This can provide a basic level of information, allowing patients to then ask more specific questions. Information giving is also important to ensure that a patient is in a position to give their consent, which will be considered later in this chapter.

WORKING WITHIN LIMITS OF COMPETENCE

Generally speaking, benefits of therapy will be achieved when hypnotherapy is delivered by well-trained therapists, working within the limits of their competence. Risks are most likely to occur when a therapist works outside his or her level of competence and provides treatment which is contraindicated and/or fails to spot conditions which require referral to another more suitable practitioner. An appropriate referral might be to another hypnotherapist who has higher-level skills (e.g. specific experience of working with children or adults who have been sexually abused), or a referral to a different specialist might be required (e.g. referral to a physician or psychiatrist). Hypnotherapists should avoid giving patients a medical diagnosis unless they are qualified to do so.

The skill of an individual practitioner will be determined by various factors. Some of these are intrinsic to the individual, such as good character, trustworthiness, and genuine warmth and empathy, whereas other skills, such as effective communication, are acquired as part of an appropriate training. One of the major ethical concerns within hypnotherapy is the variability of training and what is required to produce a competent hypnotherapist. Courses in hypnotherapy vary from short study courses over a period of weeks, to courses over a period of years. There is no agreed core curriculum, and no occupational standards which determine the competencies that a pre-registration hypnotherapist needs to be taught. This is a concern not only for therapists who work exclusively with hypnotherapy, but also for conventional practitioners, including doctors and dentists who use hypnotherapy as an adjuvant technique, e.g. for relaxation purposes. Any practitioner using hypnotherapy techniques should be appropriately trained. The failure on the part of the hypnotherapy profession to agree core competences and a standard curriculum have thwarted attempts, to date, to regulate the profession under a single professional body.

Professional, ethical and legal issues in hypnotherapy

> **BOX 3.2 Case study**
>
> A patient who has been coming for hypnotherapy treatment discloses that she has been feeling suicidal following the break-up of her marriage and talks about how she might put her plan into action.

Box 3.2 gives an example of a case where a hypnotherapist should consider a referral to a psychiatrist as a matter of urgency, as the patient not only has suicidal ideation, but has formulated an action plan. In this situation, every attempt should be made to discuss with the patient why it is felt that a referral would be helpful and any referral should be made, if at all possible, with the patient's consent, in order to maintain the patient's trust. In very rare situations where it is not possible to secure the patient's agreement, the therapist would be justified in breaching confidentiality in order to protect the patient from harm.

Avoiding harm involves working within limits of competence, and also refraining from specific techniques which are likely to cause harm. One hypnotherapy register specifically prohibits hypnotherapists from using past-life regression and exorcism or spirit-releasing techniques. Because of the concerns that hypnotherapists might abuse their position of trust when patients are in a trance (and potentially more suggestible), it is vital that a therapist using hypnotherapy techniques sets clear and firm professional boundaries. This will be discussed later in this chapter.

CONTINUOUS PROFESSIONAL DEVELOPMENT

Hypnotherapists have an ethical responsibility to keep their knowledge and skills up-to-date and to undertake continuous professional development. Many professional associations now provide CPD programmes, and undertaking CPD may, in future, be a condition of registration and revalidation. CPD courses provide practitioners with useful opportunities to ensure that they have skills in areas which may not have been taught in any great detail on their course, including ethics, law, audit and research and IT skills.

SUPERVISION

Supervision provides a useful safeguard for practitioners and patients and should be seen as integral to competent, safe practice. Supervision involves the supervisee and a supervisor meeting at regular intervals to discuss matters that may arise during the supervisee's work with clients (Mackereth & Carter 2006). A range of issues may be discussed in relation to the supervisee's client work, with matters discussed treated as confidential and the anonymity of clients preserved. Supervision is one method of ensuring that high standards of ethical practice are maintained by therapists. Hypnotherapists who are registered counsellors and psychotherapists may already access supervision, but supervision can be helpful for all hypnotherapists. Unethical practice is rarely deliberate. Poor practice is more likely to originate from inadequate training, reinforced by working in isolation from peers over a period of time. Constructive supervision may provide a necessary outlet for therapists in which technical and ethical difficulties can be discussed openly, and in a supportive and non-judgemental environment.

RECORD-KEEPING

Good records are essential for effective patient care. To benefit patients, therapists need to have a clear record of the patient's clinical history, any previous treatment, and the therapist's working diagnosis. Failing to keep good records is a serious professional breach, and is frequently a subsidiary allegation against practitioners in fitness to practice cases. Hypnotherapists must comply with their legal responsibilities in relation to data protection, ensuring that at all times both computer and manual records are maintained in accordance with statutory requirements, such as the Data Protection Act 1998. Accurate records are also critical if a practitioner is sued, so that the practitioner can establish what was or was not done or said. Records should contain the following information:

- The date of the appointment
- The patient's account of how they have been since the last visit
- The therapist's observations, including physical observations and assessment
- Any additional comments by the patient, including disagreement with the practitioner's views
- The treatment given
- Information as to risks of therapy
- Answers to any direct questions
- Confirmation that consent has been sought and discussed
- Any information received from or given to professional colleagues, e.g. members of a multidisciplinary team.

Therapists should remember that records may be inspected by other people at some time in the future, and may even be used as evidence in court. They should never include disparaging remarks, or comments which are liable to misinterpretation at a later date.

AWARENESS OF PROFESSIONAL BOUNDARIES

Professional boundaries (Stone 2008) refer to the *limits* of the professional relationship, particularly the limit between acceptable and unacceptable behaviours. Boundaries demarcate professional relationships from other relationships, such as sexual relationships, friendships or commercial relationships. It is always the professional's responsibility to set and maintain clear boundaries (CHRE 2008). The consequences for patients when practitioners breach acceptable boundaries can be very serious, particularly when a practitioner breaches emotional and/or sexual boundaries. If reported, boundary breaches are likely to result in a professional conduct case, and extreme cases of sexual abuse, including abuse involving minors or mentally incapacitated adults, may result in prosecution and a prison sentence. Allegations of abuse against hypnotherapists have been made to advocacy organizations, relating to private and NHS practitioners.

Professional, ethical and legal issues in hypnotherapy

As part of their training, therapists should learn how to forge caring, empathetic relationships, including the safe use of touch, where this is therapeutically appropriate. Hypnotherapists should be particularly mindful around the use of touch in patients who may have a history of being sexually abused and should always document their treatments and any consent given. Practitioners should also be aware of the vulnerabilities of working from their own homes, or treating patients in the patient's home with no chaperone. Practitioners should be mindful not to put themselves in situations where their behaviour or comments may be misinterpreted.

Strong feelings and emotions do arise in therapeutic relationships, but it is the therapist's responsibility to keep the relationship on a safe, professional footing, for the patient's sake and their own sake. Therapists should anticipate that patients may sometimes act in a sexually provocative way towards them, which may or may not itself be indicative of pathology, e.g. in the case of a previously abused patient who has little experience of appropriate boundaries. If a hypnotherapist becomes aware that a patient is sexually attracted to them, he or she must take all necessary precautions not to exploit the patient's vulnerability. This may, occasionally, require the therapist to hand care over to someone else, and where it is no longer possible to continue a therapeutic relationship with a practitioner, alternative arrangements should be made to ensure that the patient's therapeutic needs can continue to be met.

It is vitally important that practitioners recognize warning signs and make sure they do not act inappropriately or in a way which a patient might misconstrue. Practitioners should avoid high-risk areas, including: the giving or receiving of gifts, inappropriate personal information disclosure, use of special or untested techniques, including intimate use of touch, and arranging appointments outside normal appointment times.

Maintaining appropriate boundaries is a significant issue in hypnotherapy, where a patient will be in a trance state for part of the consultation. The Kerr/Haslam Inquiry, which investigated the sexual abuse by two psychiatrists of multiple female patients, found that both doctors had used hypnotherapy techniques as a precursor to assaulting patients. The Inquiry noted:

> Our concern is that the use of hypnotism within the NHS is not regulated and, so far as we are aware, there is no guidance from bodies such as the GMC, the BMA or the Royal College of Psychiatrists (RCP) on when, in what circumstances, or in relation to what (if any) mental disorders, it can properly and reasonably be used.
>
> (Kerr/Haslam Inquiry 2005)

They urged the National Institute of Clinical Excellence (NICE) and Royal College of Psychiatrists to look at the efficacy of this treatment in psychiatric practice. The panel recommended that hypnotherapy, along with all other therapies used by mental health professionals should be recorded and discussed through appraisal/job plans. Trusts should have a clear evidence base and protocols for guiding the use of these treatments.

The Inquiry panel stated that hypnotherapy was not usually a therapy that would be appropriate to be used on home visits and cautioned its practice in the absence of a chaperone. The panel also recommended that the Government reconsider the need for the statutory regulation of hypnotherapy, although at the time of writing, statutory regulation for hypnotherapy has not been introduced, and is not likely to be introduced in the foreseeable future.

RESPECTING AUTONOMY

It is the duty of all healthcare practitioners to respect and promote patient autonomy. This includes, but is not limited to, respecting a patient's privacy, treating them with dignity, not being judgemental, and helping patients to make good decisions for themselves. Promoting and facilitating autonomy is particularly important for patients whose autonomy may, in some way, be diminished, e.g. by poor mental health or addiction issues. Promoting autonomy includes helping patients to make decisions for themselves and not allowing them to become reliant on the therapy or the therapist. This means ensuring that therapy does not extend beyond a period that is therapeutically indicated. The duty to respect autonomy is reflected in professional practice through the key duties to obtain consent to treatment, and the duty to respect confidentiality.

CONSENT TO TREATMENT

The law recognizes that a person should not be exposed to risk unless he has voluntarily accepted that risk, on the basis of adequate information and adequate comprehension (Stone & Matthews 1996). Similarly, people should be free from being touched unless this is something they have expressly agreed to, so therapists need to get express permission to touch patients as part of treatment, and should be sure to document such agreement. In professional practice, these concerns are discussed under the heading of 'consent'.

The importance of obtaining consent cannot be overstated. Consent turns a potential battery into a legally permissible touching, and is the defence to a negligence action when a foreseeable risk arises, provided sufficient information has been given, in a form which the patient can understand. Consent cases account for a significant proportion of cases brought against CAM practitioners to professional bodies.

Failure to gain consent can give rise to two quite distinct legal actions. Where a patient has given no consent at all, an action in 'trespass' to the person may arise. In this action, there is no need to prove harm over and above the unwanted touching. Where there has been failure to give sufficient information, the action is in negligence and the complainant must be able to prove that harm resulted from the practitioner's breach of 'duty to warn'. Each will be considered below.

Trespass against the person ('battery')

Hypnotherapists should only touch patients when the patient has given consent. Up to a point, consent may be implied, where for example, a practitioner wishes to take a patient's pulse as part of a history taking, and the patient willingly holds out his or her arm. However, the use of massage under hypnosis is an example of touch which would require express consent. The use of touch within any therapy has the capacity to benefit and cause harm, particularly when working with patients with emotional issues. Although use of touch can be highly therapeutic, it can have a serious adverse impact if the touching is not expected and is not welcomed by a patient. Hypnotherapists should not make assumptions about the use of touch in their work, and this is something which should be specifically addressed in advance and negotiated with patients, with a clear explanation of any anticipated therapeutic benefit.

Therapists who touch patients without consent face the risk of a civil law action for trespass against the person, otherwise known as 'battery'. This should not be confused with criminal prosecution for assault and battery. A civil action in battery requires patients to prove:

- That a practitioner touched them without seeking their permission
- That the practitioner touched them even though they expressly refused permission
- That the practitioner had given the patient so little information that the patient didn't even understand in broad terms what was proposed.

But because the purpose of an action for battery is to protect people from unwanted interference, there is no need to prove harm over and above the unwanted touching in an action for battery.

Duty to provide information

Practitioners have a duty to inform patients of the risks involved in hypnotherapy. Practitioners should remember that even though what they are doing may seem very commonplace and unexceptional to them, a patient may have no idea even what is involved in hypnotherapy. In order to be able to consent to treatment, three elements need to be in place. Patients need to be given enough information, in a form they can understand, to make meaningful decisions; their decision to receive treatment must be voluntary; and they must be mentally competent to give their consent. Ordinarily, therapists may assume that a patient who has presented for hypnotherapy wants to receive hypnotherapy treatment. Indeed, it would be hard, if not impossible, to induce a hypnotic state in someone who did not wish to be put into a trance state. The mental capacity to consent to treatment is set at a low enough level to promote self-determination in all those capable of exercising a choice, and a patient, with or without a mental health condition, will be deemed competent to consent provided he or she is able to understand information, and hold that information for long enough to weigh it up and arrive at a decision. Adults over 18 are presumed to have the mental capacity to consent to, or refuse treatment.

For adult patients, the element of consent that is likely to be most relevant is the duty to inform. Broadly speaking, a therapist is required to disclose information that a reasonable practitioner would disclose, together with answers to any specific questions that the patient may ask. This includes information about what the therapy is likely to entail, how long the treatment itself is likely to last, any side-effects which may occur, either immediately, or subsequent to receiving therapy, and any reasons why hypnotherapy might not be suitable for that individual. In providing information, therapists should make sure that they provide sufficient time for patients to absorb information and to ask any questions. If possible, it can sometimes be helpful to impart information in a separate session before providing treatment for the first time, so that a patient can go away and read up and ask any subsequent questions if necessary. Consent is a process and not a once and for all time activity. If a practitioner is providing a series of sessions, they should check with the patient each time, and ensure that they are comfortable about receiving treatment on each and every occasion.

CONSENT AND CHILDREN

Hypnotherapists may treat children as well as adults. Working with children is a specialist area, requiring appropriate training. There are distinct ethical and legal considerations which practitioners need to be aware of, particularly in relation to consent. In law, parents usually act as proxy decision-makers on behalf of their children until they are old enough to make decisions in their own right. Legally, a child becomes an adult at 18. The notion of 'best interests' underpins parental duties. The statutory basis of decision-making for children is set out in the Children Act 1989, as amended. The key principles of the Act are that the child's welfare is paramount and children of sufficient maturity should be listened to.

Children between 16 and 18 are lawfully permitted to consent to treatment in their own right by virtue of Section 8 of the Family Reform Act 1969. It may also, however, be possible to rely on the consent of a minor who is under 16, provided they have sufficient maturity and intelligence to understand fully what hypnotherapy involves. The level of competence required to be able to consent to hypnotherapy without parental consent will be high, and in most situations, the consent of a parent should ordinarily be sought for patients under 16, even if this is not strictly necessary as a matter of law.

WORKING WITH VULNERABLE ADULTS

Hypnotherapists require appropriate competencies to work with vulnerable adults, including patients with mental health conditions. As stated, the fact that a patient has been diagnosed with a mental disorder or has mental health problems does not, of itself, render them unable to consent to treatment, and hypnotherapy may be a useful adjunctive therapy to patients receiving mental health treatment, detoxification, or addiction services. All adults will be able to consent provided they are able to make decisions on their own behalf. In law this requires the following (see Box 3.3):

BOX 3.3 Elements of decision-making

An adult is competent (i.e. has capacity) to consent to treatment if he or she can:
- Understand the information needed to make the decision
- Retain the information for long enough to make the decision
- Weigh up the information given to make a reasoned decision
- Be able to communicate his or her decision.

Practitioners should be mindful to work within the limits of their competence, and should recognize the need to refer to another practitioner, as appropriate. Practitioners should also be aware of the contraindications to treatment in working with vulnerable patients, and should, wherever possible, consult with other members of the patient's healthcare team. Practitioners working in an NHS-based service must also make sure that they comply with any relevant protocols and guidelines.

REGRESSION TECHNIQUES AND RISKS OF WORKING WITH PATIENTS WHO HAVE BEEN SEXUALLY ABUSED

Some hypnotherapists use regression techniques, and claim to be able to regress adults to be able to remember childhood memories. The use of this technique, which may have therapeutic application if carefully practised, has particular risks in relation to patients who have been sexually abused. Hypnotherapy may provoke memories of earlier sexual or other abuse. A debate has arisen around so-called 'false memories', and the validity of memories, particularly of sexual abuse, elicited by such techniques. Alleged perpetrators of sexual abuse have used 'false memory syndrome' as a defence in criminal actions. The mental health charity, MIND, notes:

> If the hypnotized subject believes that forgotten material ought to be recoverable, there is a tendency for memories of similar events, and creative fantasy material, to take the place of true memory. This distorted version of events is then believed as though it actually occurred and is known as false memory. Actively encouraging clients to produce specific memories, particularly of sexual abuse as children, is an extremely controversial procedure, which has been condemned by the majority of hypnotherapists as being dangerous.

> (MIND 2008)

The concern is that the debate around false memories, and those who elicit them, may divert attention from the significant prevalence of child sexual abuse, under-reporting, and difficulties in securing redress, which leads many people to experience mental health problems as children and in later life. The Code of Ethics of the Register for Evidence-Based Hypnotherapy and Psychotherapy states:

> All Therapists shall undertake to use due care and diligence to avoid the implantation or encouragement of any false memories in the client. Where memory recovery through regression, or similar techniques, is employed, [therapists shall undertake] to ensure at the earliest possible stage that the client is aware that experiences while in a suggestible state, or in a state of altered attention, are not necessarily accurate representations of the client's past. To base their theory and practice with regard to recovered memories on current, credible, and mainstream scientific research on the psychology of memory.

> (Register for Evidence-Based Hypnotherapy and Psychotherapy, Code of Ethics)

CONFIDENTIALITY

Another facet of respecting patient autonomy is the duty to respect patient's confidences. People cannot make their own choices and control their lives if they cannot control who has access to personal health information about

BOX 3.4 Scenario

A local newspaper telephones you about a famous patient who has successfully given up recreational drugs using a combination of hypnotherapy and acupuncture, both received from you. They want to interview you about your interesting work.

them. Therapists have a duty to respect patient information and should safeguard patient notes accordingly. Confidentiality should be respected, so far as possible, when discussing patients with professional colleagues, and anonymity should be preserved when a case is discussed for the purposes of education or research.

Confidentiality is one of the cornerstones of healthcare relationships. Patients will be asked for a lot of information about themselves, including potentially sensitive, personal information in the course of history taking and treatment. Patients impart this information in the context of a relationship of trust. Patients believe that the information they have conveyed will only be used in their best interests to allow a practitioner to reach a diagnosis and decide on treatment. Patients assume (not always correctly) that information will only be divulged with their express consent. Consider the scenario given in Box 3.4. This case highlights how important it is that not only hypnotherapists maintain confidentiality, but also ensure that confidentiality is maintained by any practice staff they may employ. In this example, it would be a breach of confidentiality even to confirm whether the person was or was not receiving treatment, without their permission. Famous patients are no different from other patients in that they deserve to have personal information about themselves and any treatment regimen kept confidential. A historic legal case established the fact that public interest disclosures, discussed below, should be limited in scope and that there is a difference between genuine public interest and what the public is interested in. The reason that it would be inappropriate to discuss the patient in the context of your work is that in doing so, you are not acting in the patient's best interests, and by breaching their confidences, you may well be harming them. Countervailing justifications, such as being able to generate publicity about effective therapeutic techniques, or generating business do not alter the underlying principle that information is held for the benefit of the patient, and must be protected accordingly.

The duty of confidentiality is not absolute, however, and most Codes of Ethics recognize certain limited exceptions to this duty. Exceptions arise, rarely, when disclosure is required to protect the patient or to protect third parties; when disclosure is required in the public interest; or when disclosure is required by a court of law. Patients may assume that they will divulge certain information when in a trance state. Accordingly, hypnotherapists should make it clear that they cannot offer an absolute duty of confidentiality. Consider the example in Box 3.5:

BOX 3.5 Case study

A man in his late 30s has come to you for help with anger management. He has recently lost his job and is responsible for child care while his wife goes out to work. He reveals during history taking that he has lashed out at his children on several occasions and is afraid that he will do it again.

Health professionals are under a statutory duty to report abuse, and a hypnotherapist, working in the National Health Service, even on a part-time basis, is likely to fall within this category. In other situations, practitioners should follow the Government's guidance set out in: *Every Child Matters* (HM Government 2006). In the above case, the practitioner has to make a decision as to whether the harm that the patient describes is sufficiently serious to merit a referral. If the patient, on enquiry, has not physically harmed his children, then it may be appropriate to explore his anger issues as part of a therapeutic regimen. However, if the therapist is told that a child or children are suffering, or at risk of suffering significant harm, they should write down everything which has given rise to the concern. The practitioner should alert the local authority's social services department or the police. If a suspicion of child abuse arises in the context of treating a child, therapists should remember that criminal proceedings might follow, so they should avoid asking the child leading questions which might undermine a prosecution, and they should not raise their concerns directly with the parent or any potential perpetrator. Where a practitioner reports suspected abuse by telephone, this should be followed-up in writing within 48 hours.

In the event of a follow-up investigation, CAM practitioners should provide relevant information to children's social care or the police about the child or family members as required. In such circumstances, a breach of confidential information will ordinarily be justified on the basis of public interest, or where a practitioner is asked by a court to provide such information. Practitioners who have concerns about this should contact their professional body or insurer for advice. This situation highlights one of the rare times when confidentiality may be breached, namely, where there are child protection issues.

Information about a patient may also legitimately be shared with other members of a multidisciplinary team on a 'need to know' basis. It is important that hypnotherapists working in integrated settings make this clear to patients. A hypnotherapist who is seeing a patient in private practice should not ordinarily contact a patient's GP or physician without the patient's consent and even when they work as part of a team, they should discuss any proposed disclosure with their patient.

RESPONDING CONSTRUCTIVELY TO COMPLAINTS

Wherever possible, hypnotherapists should strive to ensure that patient dissatisfactions, should they arise, be dealt with at a local level, without escalating to a formal complaint. Hypnotherapists, like all practitioners, may respond defensively if they are complained about, but should try to see complaints as a positive opportunity to learn and improve their practice. Most patients are grateful for the care they receive and find it hard to initiate a complaint. Accordingly, when a complaint is lodged, it is usually because the patient feels that he or she has a legitimate grievance, so it is important to ensure that they feel heard. Where necessary and appropriate, therapists should facilitate patients bringing a complaint and direct them to advocacy sources if necessary and appropriate. Most complaints escalate because of poor communication, including poor handling of a complaint itself. Hypnotherapists working within a hospital or clinic should familiarize themselves with any relevant complaints procedures.

REPORTING UNPROFESSIONAL PRACTICE OF COLLEAGUES

Most professional codes of ethics now recognize a specific ethical responsibility for therapists not only to act ethically themselves, but to speak out if they become aware of professional colleagues who are acting in an unprofessional manner. This is particularly important in relation to environments where vulnerable clients are treated, as they may be less able to vocalize complaints on their own behalf. Hypnotherapists working in hospital or clinic environments should familiarize themselves with reporting policies and protocols, and should record their concerns in the appropriate manner.

CURRENT REGULATORY STATUS OF HYPNOTHERAPY

Professional regulation is one of the principle mechanisms through which quality control of health professionals is exercised. The purpose of regulation is to protect the public by ensuring that a profession has high standards of training, practice and ethics. A regulatory system sets professional standards – what can reasonably be expected of a therapist – and takes action against therapists who fall below the standards expected of them. The main functions of regulation are set out in Box 3.6.

Because the purpose of regulation is to protect the public, it is important that any register is easily accessible, and shows clearly who is appropriately qualified and registered and who is not. Public protection is enhanced when there is only one register per profession so that members of the public and employers are not confused.

BOX 3.6 Key functions of regulation

- *Setting educational standards* for pre-registration training and accrediting schools to provide training
- *Maintaining a register* of qualified practitioners who meet those standards
- Issuing *guidance on ethics* and professional standards
- Operating procedures to take *action against practitioners whose practice* (*'fitness to practice'*) *is impaired*, for reasons of conduct, competence or poor health.

There is an important link between regulatory standards expected of professionals and the law. If a practitioner is sued, the court, in deciding an action in negligence, looks at the standards expected of a reasonable practitioner. These are the standards set down by the professional body in its codes of ethics (modified, potentially, by custom and practice). They help to give the court a baseline to determine whether the practitioner's actions fall within professionally accepted norms. This is why it is vital that all hypnotherapists know what their code of ethics states and work within it at all times. Therapists who deviate from their code need to be able to justify why they have acted as they have and may be held to account before a professional tribunal.

Hypnotherapy is currently a voluntary self-regulated profession. This means that there is no legal or statutory compulsion for practitioners to be registered with any registering or accredited body, and there is no legal protection of the title 'hypnotherapist'. People can call themselves a hypnotherapist with varying degrees of training and competence, which is why it is important that the patient ensures that the practitioner they are consulting has received appropriate training and is registered with a suitable body.

Registering bodies in the UK include: the British Hypnotherapy Association, the Hypnotherapy Association UK, the National Register of Hypnotherapists and Psychotherapists (NRHP), the Register for Evidence Based Hypnotherapy and Psychotherapy and the British Association of Medical Hypnosis. The UK Confederation of Hypnotherapy Organizations is an umbrella organization with organizational members (see Useful Resources). Additionally, therapists may be trained in another healthcare discipline and be regulated by a separate regulatory body. This will include counsellors and psychotherapists using hypnotherapy techniques.

SUMMARY

Despite calls for hypnotherapy to be statutorily regulated, this is unlikely to happen in the foreseeable future. Hypnotherapy is not one of the therapies included in the new federal voluntary self-regulating body for complementary and alternative therapists, the Complementary and Natural Healthcare Council (CHNC), established in April 2008. As noted by the House of Lords Select Committee in 2000, regulation of hypnotherapy has been particularly elusive. Until such time as hypnotherapy is able to establish a single register, and coherent standards of training and practice, in order to protect patients, it behoves individual practitioners to make themselves aware of their ethical and legal responsibilities, and to ensure that they work within the protocols of any employing institution. Practitioners should ensure that they are both appropriately registered and carry professional indemnity insurance and should be ready and willing to explain to prospective patients and employers, their therapeutic orientation, the nature of their training and qualifications, and any CPD or supervision they regularly undertake.

REFERENCES

Council for Healthcare Regulatory Excellence (CHRE), 2008. Clear sexual boundaries between healthcare professionals and patients: responsibilities of healthcare professionals. Council for Healthcare Regulatory Excellence, London.

HM Government, 2006. What to do if you're worried a child is being abused. Online Available: www.everychildmatters.gov.uk/_files/FD21D51F594298457CF64BE9CDF6F179.pdf.

House of Lords, 2000. Complementary and alternative medicine: House of Lords Science and Technology Select Committee Sixth Report. Online. Available: www.publications.parliament.uk/pa/ld199900/ldselect/ldsctech/123/12301.htm.

Kerr/Haslam Inquiry, 2005. HM Government, Command 6640, July.

Mackereth, P.A., Carter, A., 2006. Professional and potent practice. In: Mackereth, A., Carter, A. (Eds.), Massage and bodywork: adapting therapies for cancer care. Churchill Livingstone, Edinburgh.

MIND, Online. Available: www.mind.org.uk/Information/Factsheets/Treatments+and+drugs/Hypnotherapy.htm.

Register for Evidence-Based Hypnotherapy and Psychotherapy. Online. Available: http://www.rebhp.org/codeofethics.htm.

Stone, J., 2008. Respecting professional boundaries: what CAM practitioners need to know. Complement. Ther. Clin. Pract. 14, 2–7.

Stone, J., Matthews, J., 1996. Complementary medicine and the law. Oxford University Press, Oxford.

FURTHER READING

Beauchamp, T., Childress, J., 1994. Principles of biomedical ethics, fourth ed. Oxford University Press, Oxford.

Hunter, M., Struve, J., 1998. The ethical use of touch in psychotherapy. Sage, London.

Stone, J., 2002. An ethical framework for complementary and alternative therapists. Routledge, London.

USEFUL RESOURCES

British Society of Clinical Hypnosis, www.bsch.org.uk.

Medical School Hypnosis Association (MSHA), www.mhsa.org.uk.

National Council for Hypnotherapy, www.hypnotherapists.org.uk.

The Hypnotherapy Association, www.thehypnotherapyassociation.co.uk.

The National Register of Hypnotherapists and Psychotherapists (NRHP), www.nrhp.co.uk.

The Register for Evidence Based Hypnotherapy and Psychotherapy, www.rebhp.org.

The UK Confederation of Hypnotherapy Organizations, www.ukcho.co.uk.

Professional, ethical and legal issues in hypnotherapy

4 Research and hypnotherapy interventions

Graeme Donald

CHAPTER OUTLINE

This chapter provides the reader with an overview of how research links into hypnotherapy practice. It examines the body of evidence supporting the use of hypnotherapy in a variety of settings, offering a selection of published studies to be considered. The reader will be introduced to concepts such as evidence-based practice and aspects of the research process. Research into complementary and alternative medicine (CAM) interventions, such as hypnotherapy, is an evolving discipline and some of the issues surrounding this topic are touched upon. The author has included recommendations for the direction of future research projects investigating hypnotherapy.

© 2010 Elsevier Ltd.
DOI: 10.1016/B978-0-7020-3082-6.00006-X

Research
Evidence-based practice
Methodology
Qualitative and quantitative approaches

INTRODUCTION

Since the concept and practice of hypnosis was defined in the late 1800s, evolving from Mesmerism, it has been of interest to those working in the medical and psychological professions. Practitioners have been able to see the benefits available from suspending the critical faculties of the conscious mind in a number of different settings. One important question needs to be asked however – does it work? Consumers may seek out hypnotherapy on a private basis for a variety of reasons, including ego strengthening, anxiety management or behavioural changes. In this context, the reputation that hypnotherapy has earned itself may be enough for an individual to part with their money. It is not so simple if it is to be offered as a service that is funded by public money. Healthcare providers, such as hospitals and primary care trusts, are ultimately accountable to the taxpayer to ensure that the services they provide are value for money. Thus decisions that are made regarding service provision have to cover whether it is needed or wanted, whether the services are going to deliver and will they be cost-effective.

EVIDENCE-BASED PRACTICE

The ethos of evidence-based practice is a simple one; it involves the application of best practice and the best use of resources. From its rise in the UK in the early 1990s, it has spread to become a global phenomenon and is now the foundation of UK health policy (Reynolds 2000). It has led to the creation of the National Institute for Health and Clinical Excellence (NICE), an independent body responsible for providing guidance on the promotion of good health and the treatment of ill health. This guidance aims to achieve consistency across health services, ensuring they are up-to-date and that they provide good value to health consumers. Sometimes politically sensitive, the sad matter of fact is that the publicly funded health services do not have endless reserves to draw upon and so resources must be used as best as possible, based on the evidence available. This is why, if CAM interventions like hypnotherapy are to be further integrated into the NHS, the need for high-quality research evidence must be met.

It is not just health providers and consumers that want the evidence to be widely available but also practitioners. Doctors, nurses and therapists, most of whom were drawn to their discipline with a desire to help, need confirmation that their actions are having a positive effect on the patient. Indeed, many CAM training courses now provide a programme of research within their syllabus which may include awareness of what the evidence says, how to find it and on the research process itself.

The House of Lords Science and Technology Report (2000) identified the lack of high-quality CAM research available and recommended that work be done to ensure that such practices be exposed to the same level of scientific rigour as conventional medicine. The report classified different therapies into three groups and placed hypnotherapy in Group 2 alongside practices like massage, aromatherapy and meditation. While satisfied that therapies in this category provide comfort and can help to complement medical treatments, the report nonetheless acknowledges the lack of a scientific basis from where they are practiced. It further recommends that structures for regulation and education are strengthened and that the evidence base is developed to underpin practice.

REASONS FOR ENGAGING IN RESEARCH

The idea of conducting a research project may seem a daunting one for a hypnotherapist. Essentially, however, research is simply the acquisition of knowledge. This can be obtained through a variety of means:

- Tradition – 'this is the way that it has always been done'
- Expert opinion – listening to the teachings of accepted experts in their fields and the wisdom they have gained through experience. This could include editorials from respected figures such as Ericksson and Hilgard
- Trial and error – practitioners reflecting on their practice, what worked and what did not and adapting for the next time
- Historical analysis – examining a range of sources to provide a history of the development of practice and philosophy in a given field
- Science – applying a logical and systematic framework to the measurement and observation of a phenomenon.

A therapist's belief that hypnotherapy works may come from observing changes in their clients, this may be a sufficient basis for their ongoing individual practice. Equally, consumers of hypnotherapy may experience the benefits and not require that it be proven scientifically to them. Anecdotal evidence can provide interesting 'cases' to reflect upon. Indeed, further understanding of the application and effects of hypnotherapy can be gained by analysing the processes and outcomes for one individual. Standing alone, however, these case reports are not enough to widen the scope of practice for hypnotherapy. Ozturk (2006) reported on the case of a woman undergoing a cholecystectomy, the removal of her gall bladder. The surgery was conducted with the patient being inducted into trance but without the use of any medication. Remaining pain-free, she was conscious during the operation and was eventually discharged earlier than the accepted norm. While a case like this fires the imagination, it does not provide enough evidence to justify replacing general anaesthesia with hypnosis in similar cases. Science demands that studies are easily replicated and it may be difficult to reproduce the conditions that were in place in the previous example. The next patient may have low hypnotic susceptibility or may experience a spontaneous emergence from trance. In either case, the resulting effects may be dramatic and potentially devastating.

The aforementioned case study cited by Ozturk (2006) illustrates the need to identify variables involved in treatment, to measure them, control them and to ascertain the effects that they have on the treatment as a whole. Until quantified, the effect of variables on treatment outcomes is unknown. Examples of such variables include hypnotic susceptibility, the rapport between therapist and client, length of treatment, suggestions used and the context in which hypnotherapy is employed.

AREAS FOR RESEARCH

As mentioned earlier, the primary question that research into hypnotherapy should answer is 'does it work'? Delving deeper, other questions quickly come to the fore:

- When does it work?
- Who does it work with?
- How does it work?
- Does it work better than existing treatments?
- Does it enhance existing treatments?
- Is it simply a placebo effect?

It is easy to see that no one study can possibly answer all the questions posed. An enthusiastic hypnotherapist or potential researcher may want to 'prove' that hypnotherapy works in one fell swoop; not only is that impractical but it is impossible. Not only is hypnotherapy a complex inter-vention, but the demographic differences (diagnosis, reasons for attending, expectations, etc.) among the patients who use it will also vary widely. The budding researcher needs to identify potential areas of interest (Box 4.1), to refine the question that they want to answer, to plan the most appropriate way they can answer it and, most importantly, to ensure that their question has not been answered satisfactorily by someone else. It would be a waste of time, effort and money to conduct a study if there already existed one of sufficient quality that showed significant effects. However, if a previous study had been conducted and the question posed had not been answered definitively, then a follow-up study would be feasible.

BOX 4.1 Potential areas of investigation

- Evidence of the safety and efficacy of hypnotherapy in a variety of situations
- Exploration of the reasons that people seek hypnotherapy treatments
- Description of what people experience when in trance and the value that they attach to it
- Mechanism of operation
- Survey of the preconceptions that people hold of hypnotherapy
- Development of new and appropriate research strategies
- Comparison against other available treatments
- Evaluation of services offering hypnotherapy
- Investigation into the quality, variability and accessibility of training
- Identification of how susceptibility affects outcome.

HIERARCHY OF EVIDENCE

With so many varied options when deciding on a particular research design, it is worthwhile to give the following brief synopsis of the two categories that they fall into.

QUANTITATIVE STUDIES

Quantitative studies follow the traditional, scientific method that involves employing a set of processes to obtain information. Grounded in positivist philosophy, the quantitative researcher might believe that an absolute reality exists beyond human perception and that this reality can be measured. The results of a quantitative design will often be reduced to a numerical form and be analysed using statistical procedures to ascertain whether or not a relationship exists in reality. Strict adherence to pre-specified procedures and objectivity are not just seen as desirable in such a study, they are a necessity. Qualitative researchers are interested in the human experience and attempt to explore it directly. In this naturalistic philosophy, reality is not seen as an immutable fact but rather that multiple realities exist, mentally constructed by the individual. The belief inherent in this school of thought is that a human being is too complex to be boiled down to a set of numbers and that the different dimensions of an individual's experience can be described and understood.

Randomized controlled trial (RCT) is seen as the gold standard in determining the effectiveness of a given treatment. It is seen as 'true' experimental research, attempting to translate laboratory conditions to the larger world. Participants are randomly allocated to different groups, exposed to an intervention and then the results are measured. The inclusion of a control group provides a benchmark for the intervention to be tested against and members of the control group could be exposed to an alternative treatment or to no treatment. Variables that are known or suspected to affect the outcome are called confounders and they are controlled as much as possible so that the results only represent the effects of the intervention used. Ideally, an RCT would be double-blinded, i.e. neither researcher nor subject would know which intervention has been provided. In practice, this is only possible for drug trials, where the subject would be unaware whether the tablet they have taken is the active treatment or a placebo pill. In CAM research, this is impossible; it would be hard to imagine that someone would be unaware of whether they were receiving hypnotherapy or massage as part of a research trial. It is possible, however, for a researcher to blind themselves to the allocation of subjects within a trial and this is referred to as a single-blinded trial. Quasi-experimental designs encompass most of the features of the RCT but not all. It may be that there is no control group or no random allocation and so this lack of precision is why such designs are secondary to the RCT.

QUALITATIVE STUDIES

Qualitative studies are seen as more person-centred and attempt to grasp the essence of what has transpired, from the perspective of the patient. Phenomenology is a tradition in qualitative research, founded by Husserl and Heidegger that lends itself well to investigating CAM interventions like hypnotherapy.

> **BOX 4.2 Hierarchy of evidence**
>
> **High quality**
> - Systematic reviews/meta-analyses of randomized controlled trials
> - Randomized controlled trials
> - Experimental designs
>
> **Moderate quality**
> - Cohort studies
> - Case control/case series
>
> **Low quality**
> - Expert opinion
> - Observational studies
> - Qualitative studies
>
> Adapted from Sackett et al (2000).

Used a great deal in the field of psychology, it focuses on the meaning of people's lived experiences. Broadly speaking, it would involve interviewing participants after receiving a hypnotherapy session, looking to answer questions regarding what they experienced during treatment, how they felt about it and how their perception of the focus of their treatment had been affected. Qualitative researchers see the subjective nature of their work as its strength. They believe the value that an individual derives from a therapy can affect the way they feel about themselves and the way they live their lives. It would be difficult for an RCT to quantify, observe and measure such concepts.

Box 4.2 outlines the accepted hierarchy of evidence within the medical sciences, adapted from Sackett et al (2000), which forms a component of NHS research and development policy. It is easy to see that quantitative methodologies dominate the classification of acceptable evidence and thus the research priorities to affect change in service provision. Historically, clinicians have been interested in whether or not a treatment works and whether the effect can be measured. And so there exists a potential conflict as hypnotherapists may be more interested in how their clients feel about the treatment and how it has affected the way they live their lives. Such questions naturally draw themselves toward a qualitative design and although results may be compelling, parts of the medical establishment may well consider them substandard when compared with the results of a well-designed RCT.

CAM RESEARCH ISSUES

The central problem surrounding the research of complementary therapies is borne in the opposite nature of two paradigms. Conventional medicine values empirical science while complementary therapists value the individual perspectives of holistic methods. For example, some complementary therapists claim that quantitative research methods are not appropriate to evaluate therapies (Tonelli & Callahan 2003). However, many mainstream scientists argue that CAM interventions should be exposed to the same rigorous processes as conventional medicine, particularly if they are to be integrated into mainstream healthcare (Lewith 2003). Lewith argues that subjecting therapies, like hypnotherapy, to conventional research methodologies helps to answer questions of clinical significance. It is also important to acknowledge practitioners' claims that quantitative research dissects their therapy and do not hold true, particularly when RCTs have been conducted to measure the effects of interventions like psychotherapy, prayer and quality of life, all of which are arguably subjective by nature. Vincent and Furnham (1998) suggest that the first question to be posed should be whether or not the therapy has a beneficial effect on a disease. However, they caution that such objective measures may not be as important to patients themselves as more subjective concepts like their quality of life.

And so the debate over the most appropriate forms of research for complementary therapies carries on. The most contentious issue here is whether RCTs are as useful at evaluating hypnotherapy as they are at evaluating the effect that a new medicine has. The question becomes whether the traditional RCT should be used, whether it can be customized to reflect the holistic techniques applied through hypnotherapy or whether it should be discarded and replaced with more appropriate methods. The problem with discarding the RCT for hypnotherapy research is that, for example if replaced largely by phenomenological studies, then no matter how consistent and compelling the results might be, they would still be classified as Tier 3 studies within the hierarchy of evidence. It would be very unlikely that the accumulation of this type of evidence would lead to changes in healthcare provision without being supported by what is viewed as stronger evidence of experimental designs. Approaching a research problem within the traditional RCT design, however, while ticking the boxes for strong evidence, may overlook some of the possible effects of the hypnotherapy. As a treatment, it is holistic, focusing on a variety of psychological resources that already exist within the client and helps the client access these when they need them. The complexity of such a treatment may well be lost if conditions are tightly controlled within a trial and a standardized hypnotherapy script will probably not be as effective as one that would be customized to the individual. In practice, a hypnotherapist would not assist with reducing anxiety in two clients using identical strategies and so, in adopting a singular strategy during an RCT, the research may not reflect practice effectively.

Another question in the creation of a RCT is: *what type of intervention to compare the hypnotherapy treatment against?* As discussed earlier, the inclusion of a control group provides a benchmark for comparison and a researcher may want to think carefully about the control intervention. The first option would be a 'no treatment' group, but there are a number of concerns associated with this study design. Critics of CAM interventions argue that the therapeutic effects are derived from the placebo response that is that the patient believes that the treatment will work and it is this expectation that creates the effect, rather than the therapy itself. Furthermore, to withhold treatment from members of the control group can raise ethical issues; the researcher may be seen as withholding a potentially effective treatment, which contradicts the healthcare tenet of 'doing no harm' (see Ch. 3). Common practice is to replace no treatment with 'standard care', which is the medical care that the participant would have received if they were not part of the research trial. The problem of how to control for the placebo effect still arises. Recent studies have included an attention-control group to mediate the placebo effect. A member of the research team would counsel each member of the group, discussing whatever concerns were raised but avoiding any suggestions. To achieve parity across groups, the attention session would last for the same length of time as the hypnotherapy session. More recently, Gholamrezaei and Emami (2008) have proposed an alternative placebo control that remains to be tested. They recognize that attention control does not involve hypnosis and that even the mention of the treatment may elicit a response from members of the active treatment group. They suggest 'neutral hypnosis' as a credible form of placebo control – that is exposing participants to induction and trance deepening but working with only non-therapeutic imagery, such as the sea or a garden, rather than using suggestions designed to enhance mental or physical health. Recognizing that such imagery does not seem to have a therapeutic effect, they consider that 'neutral hypnosis' provides a better basis of comparison as both treatments can be labelled as hypnotherapy.

There is a growing consensus among researchers that, rather than remaining entrenched in their respective camps, there are ways to draw on the strengths of quantitative and qualitative methods to devise sound mixed method approaches to CAM research. Block et al (2004) postulate that RCTs are necessary in researching CAM interventions but that the inclusion of qualitative data provides useful information like functionality, sleep and the perceptions of illness and intervention. Verhoef et al (2005) concur and go on to suggest that including qualitative aspects into the rigour of a controlled trial can prove most useful. Comparing the differences in perceptions between members of trial groups may provide even more data to better evaluate CAM interventions. Furthermore, adapting an RCT can create a 'pragmatic trial' that allows the inclusion of customized treatments based on individual needs but within the parameters of the RCT. Broom and Adams (2007) further advocate the mixed method approach and suggest a number of frameworks that may be adopted in future research (Box 4.3).

THE RESEARCH PROCESS

The potential researcher must begin by identifying their area of interest and refining it, by asking what context they wish to explore hypnotherapy, what methods they want to evaluate and in what group of people. A clearly defined area is a necessity – the wider the scope, the less direction the researcher will have. While exploring the options, it is important to consider whether there will be practical implications of the findings and, to be pragmatic, whether there will be funding available. Novice researchers often find it difficult to secure funding on their own. It would be advantageous to the development and submission of proposal for funding to team up with an experienced researcher(s) who has already successfully completed and published research work. To make a project viable, funding should encompass all aspects of the study, which includes researchers' time, stationery, participant expenses, room hire and consultancy fees. It is the researcher's responsibility to identify all associated costs of the study and to include them in a detailed costing within the proposal being submitted to the funding body.

BOX 4.3 Potential frameworks for future CAM research

Diary analysis
Provides a window into the daily, lived experiences of patients. It can track the evolution of patient perceptions of their health over time. Participants need to be committed to the study to maintain the effort necessary for diary-keeping over a long period of time.

Focus groups
Regularly used in social science research. Combines interviewing and observation of participants to obtain a lot of information in a short period of time. Analysis of group dynamics can also provide useful data.

Action research
A research style, rather than method, where the researcher works with and for a client group, rather than working on them. Creating solutions to problems is the focus of this work and the client group leads the researcher. Increasingly used within healthcare settings.

Delphi method
An iterative process that involves clarifying inconsistencies in published studies by attaining a consensus among experts within the field. While expert opinion is low on the hierarchy of evidence, a collective opinion within the context of published studies provides more influential evidence.

Adapted from Broom and Adams (2007).

From identifying the research problem, time must be taken to carefully formulate the research question. This is arguably the most important point in the process; the entire basis for the subsequent project can be drawn from the research question. It should be concise, direct, understandable to others, and should stem from the identified area of interest. During a trial, the researcher should be able to return to the question to help clarify the central issues. The right question will give clear direction for the study, it will help determine the study design, identify the population to be recruited from, what, when and how the data need to be collected, and importantly the analysis required to answer the question poised.

The Research Governance Framework (DoH 2005) provides guidelines on how to conduct ethical research and is a must-read for all researchers. Essentially, its first purpose is to protect the human rights of those who agree to take part in a study. In the early 1900s, many studies were conducted that included dubious and sometimes scandalous methods. Early psychological studies into brain function included manually stimulating areas of the brain in a fully conscious subject and monitoring the effects. Clearly such behaviour would be completely unacceptable in modern times. The framework is rooted in the protection of the four main ethical principles of modern healthcare – autonomy, justice, doing good and doing no harm (Seedhouse 1998). Any researcher should be completely honest with themselves when reflecting on the ethical concerns of their study design, especially given the large proportion of potentially vulnerable patients that hypnotherapists work with. Any research project that is proposed which requires access to users of the NHS will be required to submit an application to a Research Ethics Committee (REC). These committees are notoriously difficult to please, given their massive responsibility, and so care should be taken to adequately follow the guidelines available before reaching this point.

CONTEMPORARY HYPNOTHERAPY RESEARCH

Since the advent of evidence-based practice and recent moves towards the integration of complementary therapies into mainstream healthcare, there has been a growth in research work undertaken to demonstrate the benefits that hypnotherapy can offer. Table 4.1 gives a selection of this work and, although this list is not exhaustive, it shows the effects that hypnotherapy can have. The wide spectrum of these studies reinforces the versatility of hypnotherapy and its potential to be integrated into a variety of healthcare settings.

MEDICAL PROCEDURES

Lang et al (2000) identified the increasing trend of replacing open surgery under general anaesthesia with procedures guided by radiological scans. They became interested in the beneficial effects that hypnotherapy could have for patients undergoing such procedures. Patients were randomized into three groups receiving either the standard care for the institution, structured attentive listening or self-hypnotic relaxation. Each of the three interventions provided adhered to manuals to achieve standardization across all participants. Patients had access to nurse-administered intravenous sedation and analgesia upon their request and were asked to self-rate their pain and anxiety on a verbal scale from 0 to 10 every 15 minutes. Participants' vital signs were monitored throughout using automated systems. The trial found that pain increased over time in the attention and standard care groups but remained flat in the hypnosis group, while drug use was significantly higher in the standard care group. Anxiety decreased in time across all three groups but more steeply in the hypnosis group. It is unclear whether the nature of the procedures was equivalent across groups but the authors noted that procedure time was less in the hypnosis group, suggesting that a future analysis into cost-effectiveness may be possible. Interestingly, only one participant from the hypnosis group became unstable during the procedures, less than in the other groups. This may indicate that an aspect of hypnotherapy leads to optimal functioning, even during invasive medical procedures. This may be an area of interest in future studies. Lang et al (2008) continued their investigations with a similarly designed trial on patients undergoing tumour treatments. Findings showed that members of the hypnosis group, again, experienced lower levels of pain and anxiety and needed less analgesia. The trial had to be discontinued on ethical grounds before conclusion however, as members of the attention-control group were experiencing a disturbingly high rate of intra-procedural adverse events. All patients were successfully treated but the trial was halted to protect the safety of participants. The authors suggest that care must be

Table 4.1 *Hypnotherapy research 2000–2008*

Study	Objective	Design	Outcome measures	Results	Comments
Lang et al (2000)	To test non-pharmacological behavioural adjuncts as efficient safe means of reducing discomfort and adverse effects during medical procedures	RCT ($n = 241$) 1. Standard care intraoperatively 2. Structured attention 3. Self-hypnotic relaxation	Pain and anxiety verbal analogue scales every 15 min Use of analgesia	Pain increased with time in standard and attention groups but remained flat in hypnosis group. Anxiety decreased more in hypnosis group than others Analgesia use significantly higher in standard group. Less intraoperative adverse events in hypnosis group	Clinicians blinded to attention/hypnosis allocation Hypnotic script adapted during trial for logistical reasons Analgesia administered at patient request Procedures not stratified across groups
Martin et al (2001)	To evaluate how hypnotic preparation affects labour processes and birth outcomes of pregnant adolescents	RCT ($n = 42$) 1. Hypnosis group 2. Supportive counselling	Medication use Complications Surgical intervention Hospital stay Neonatal ICU admissions	Hypnosis group experienced significantly less complications, shorter hospital stays and needed no surgical intervention compared with 12 in counselling group. There were non-significant reductions in medication use and neonatal ICU admissions	Low external validity due to narrow population Small sample size Inclusion of standard care group would be useful
Gonsalkorale et al (2002)	An evaluation of a hospital-based hypnotherapy service for people with irritable bowel syndrome	Audit ($n = 250$) Patients received 12 hypnotherapy sessions over a 3-month period	Questionnaires given pre- and post-treatment measuring IBS symptoms, extracolonic features, quality of life, anxiety and depression	Hypnotherapy improved IBS symptoms and extra-colonic features. 78% of patients had improved bowel habits while 9% suffered a deterioration. Quality of life, anxiety and depression were significantly improved	Improved IBS scores directly correlated to improved quality of life, anxiety and depression; 18 participants withdrew before all 12 sessions but were included in statistical analysis No follow-up Little effect for males with diarrhoea

Taylor & Ingleton (2003)	To investigate the experiences of cancer patients participating in a programme of CBT and hypnotherapy while receiving chemotherapy	Qualitative study with semi-structured interviews (n = 8)	Thematic analysis of interview transcripts	Patients reported being able to relax, sleep and cope better with fear and side-effects They felt more empowered to take control and used tools in many aspects of their lives. HCPs did not readily refer patients to the service	Participants specifically targeted for recruitment Setting's association with a hospice altered patients' perspectives Negative preconceptions of hypnosis had to be tackled
Bryant et al (2005)	To evaluate the additive effect of combining hypnosis with cognitive behavioural therapy (CBT) in the treatment of acute stress disorder (ASD)	RCT (n = 87) 1. CBT group 2. CBT-hypnosis 3. Supportive counselling (SC) CBT-hypnosis followed same protocol as CBT group but included induction and suggestions to fully engage in process	Impact of Event Scale (IES) Beck Anxiety Inventory (BAI) Beck Depression Inventory-2 (BDI-2) Clinician Administered Post-traumatic Stress Disorder Scale-2 (CAPS-2)	CBT-hypnosis group had re-experienced fewer PTSD symptoms post-treatment than CBT alone. Both groups showed significant reductions in symptoms at follow-up compared to SC	High attrition rate Researchers suggest they limited scope of clinical gains of hypnosis through the method of its employment Larger numbers may detect more differences between CBT and CBT-hypnosis
Liossi et al (2006)	To compare the efficacy of an analgesic cream with hypnosis in the relief of lumbar-puncture-induced pain and anxiety	RCT (n = 45) 1. Local anaesthetic (LA) 2. LA plus hypnosis 3. LA plus attention	Wong-Baker FACES pain rating scale Procedure behaviour checklist Stanford Hypnotic Clinical Scale for children	Children in LA plus hypnosis group experienced significantly less anticipatory anxiety, procedure-related pain and anxiety. Observers noted less overt signs of physical distress in hypnosis group	Observers were blinded to allocation Same therapist for all groups Mild deviation in therapist behaviour necessitated by children's reactions during procedure

continued

Table 4.1 *Hypnotherapy research 2000–2008—cont'd*

Study	Objective	Design	Outcome measures	Results	Comments
Saadat et al (2006)	To examine the effects of hypnosis on preoperative anxiety	RCT (*n* = 76) 1. Hypnosis group 2. Attentive listening 3. Standard care	STAI, Visual Analogue Scale (VAS) for anxiety, BP, HR at pre and post-treatment VAS on entry to operating room	Hypnosis group were significantly less anxious post-treatment, based on STAI At entry to operating room, hypnosis group reported a reduction in baseline anxiety while other groups reported an increase, based on VAS No change in BP or HR	Assessors blinded to intervention No mention of type of surgery No measurement of postoperative outcomes
Van de Vusse et al (2006)	To examine physiological and psychological effects of hypnosis on women	Quasi-experimental within-subjects repeated measures study (*n* = 30)	Heart rate Respiration rate POMS Heart rate variability (HRV)	Significant reductions in heart rate, respiration rate and HRV Significant reduction in tension–anxiety on POMS	Pilot study Narrow population Healthy participants
Duff & Nightingale (2007)	To explore the use of hypnosis to influence psychological quality of life in individuals with dementia	Pilot RCT (*n* = 18) 1. Hypnosis group 2. Discussion group 3. Standard care group	7-point Likert scale on 7 areas of quality of life (concentration, relaxation, motivation, ADLs, immediate memory, memory for significant events, socialization) Assessed by nursing staff	Hypnosis increased mean quality of life compared with discussion groups or standard care allocation Results maintained at 12-month follow-up	Assessment tool not validated Nurse assessors blinded Assessors may have applied different criteria to patients Staff reported hypnosis group were less challenging and became more active

Research and hypnotherapy interventions

	Aim	Design	Outcome measures	Results	Comments
Lang et al (2008)	To determine the effect that hypnosis and empathic attention have on pain, anxiety, drug use and adverse events during percutaneous tumour treatments	RCT (n = 201) 1. Hypnosis group 2. Attention group 3. Standard care Hypnosis group also received empathic attention	Pain and anxiety verbal analogue scales every 15 min Use of analgesia Incidence of adverse events	Hypnosis group experienced significantly less pain and anxiety compared with other groups and used less analgesia. Attention group experienced 48% adverse event rate	Unexpectedly high adverse events in attention group required trial to be discontinued Investigators also provided interventions Clinicians not blinded to allocation
Patterson & Jenkinson (2003)	To review the research on the hypnotic management of pain	Literature review	N/A	Hypnosis consistently better than standard care or attention control in acute pain Hypnosis better than standard care in chronic pain but comparable with attention controls Hypnosis not outperformed by any other interventions Evidence suggests it is a feasible intervention for acute and chronic pain	Chronic pain has more complex biopsychosocial aspects and these need to be addressed properly Few studies post-1995 Rigour of studies could be improved
Wilson et al (2006)	To systematically review the literature evaluating hypnotherapy in the management of IBS	Systematic review	N/A	18 trials and two case series were eligible Most trials showed significant benefit, internal validity was adequate Evidence suggests hypnotherapy is effective in IBS management	No data synthesis due to varied outcomes measures Hypnotherapy should be restricted to specialist centres until randomized placebo controlled trial with high internal validity is undertaken

RCT, randomized controlled trial; IBS, irritable bowel syndrome; ADLs, activities of daily living; POMS, profile of mood states; STAI, State Trait Anxiety Inventory; HR, heart rate; BP, blood pressure; PTSD, post-traumatic stress disorder; HCPs, healthcare professionals; ICU, intensive care unit.

taken in providing structured attention to ensure a lack of potentially negative suggestions. They also need to recognize that people have the capacity to go into trance spontaneously and that providing this type of intervention may prevent them from doing so. The efficacy of using attention as a safe control must be considered in light of this study for future research.

Conducting invasive medical procedures on children can be upsetting, not only for the child, but for the clinicians and for the onlooking parents. Liossi et al (2006) studied the effects that hypnosis may have in this context by conducting an RCT on children with cancer undergoing lumbar puncture. The children were randomly allocated to one of three groups which received either: (1) local anaesthetic cream, (2) attention with local anaesthetic or (3) hypnosis with local anaesthetic. Results showed that the hypnosis group experienced less anxiety before and during the procedure and less pain during the procedure. The clinicians, who were blinded to the allocation, noted that children in the hypnosis group displayed less distress during the procedure. The therapist remained constant across the groups, training the hypnosis group prior to lumbar puncture and touched the child's cheek in the treatment room to signal them to begin self-hypnosis (see Ch. 12).

Going under general anaesthetic for an operation can be stressful and managing preoperative anxiety is normally undertaken by nursing staff. Saadat et al (2006) investigated how well hypnotherapy can supplement this process. Participants were allocated to three different groups receiving a 30-minute hypnotherapy intervention, a 30-minute empathic attention session or standard institutional care. Members of the hypnosis group were significantly less anxious after receiving treatment than the attention or standard care groups. Furthermore, on entry to the operating theatre, anxiety in the hypnosis group had decreased from baseline, while the other groups experienced higher levels of anxiety. Although there was no mention of the type of surgery, which may represent a significant factor in levels of anxiety experienced, the study demonstrates that hypnotherapy may be an effective treatment in reducing preoperative anxiety, resulting in better patient experience.

IRRITABLE BOWEL SYNDROME

The hypnotherapeutic treatment of irritable bowel syndrome (IBS) has been widely studied and reported (see Ch. 13); this has led to the inception of a specialist hypnotherapy service based at the University Hospital of South Manchester. Gonsalkorale et al (2002) conducted an audit of the service's effectiveness, based on the first 250 patients. Patients were asked to complete questionnaires prior to treatment and also on conclusion of their 12 sessions of hypnotherapy, provided over a 3-month period. They were also required to practice self-hypnosis between therapy sessions. The questionnaires had been previously validated and covered IBS symptoms, extracolonic features, anxiety, depression and quality-of-life (QOL) measures. The results showed that hypnotherapy significantly improved all measures and that the improvement in IBS symptoms was correlated to a perceived improvement in QOL, anxiety and depression. Here, the causative relationship remains unclear; hypnotherapy may have ameliorated IBS symptoms leading to improvement in QOL, or, it may have directly affected QOL which, in turn, improved the patients' IBS symptoms. The only group not to improve as a result of treatment was males with a diarrhoea-predominant bowel habit.

Signifying the extent to which hypnotherapy has been studied in regard to IBS; a systematic review has been included in this overview (Wilson et al 2006). Systematic reviews are at the top of the evidence hierarchy as they search the available evidence on a given topic and include only what has met strict predetermined criteria. Analysis of each study is then undertaken using a rigorous process before a summative conclusion is reached. They involve more than one reviewer so that agreement may be achieved and that the results are not the opinion of only one person. Wilson et al (2006) searched a number of electronic databases and found 20 studies that matched the inclusion criteria; 18 trials and two case series. All papers showed that hypnotherapy had a beneficial effect on IBS symptoms. A total of 56% of the trials showed significant effects, while 83% of the controlled trials (the most methodical design) also showed significant effect. They noted that most of the studies they reviewed could have improved their internal validity and suggest this as a future area for research. They could not combine the data reviewed because the studies used a variety of outcome measures; however they conclude that the evidence suggests that hypnotherapy is an effective treatment for IBS. They go on to caution that, until a trial of high internal validity is undertaken, it should be provided only in specialist treatment centres, much like the service audited by Gonsalkorale et al (2002).

PREGNANCY

Martin et al (2001) conducted a randomized trial to investigate the effects that hypnotherapy may have on labour processes and birth outcomes in pregnant teenagers. Participants were randomized to receive either supportive counselling during the antenatal period or birth preparation while in a hypnotic state. Both groups also received the standard care for the institution. Members of the hypnosis group had a reduced hospital stay and experienced fewer complications than the control group, while none (0) of them required surgical intervention compared with 12 in the control condition. This may be linked to the increased haemodynamic stability noted by Lang et al (2000). Although not statistically significant, fewer patients used medication in the hypnosis group and less babies needed to be admitted to the neonatal ICU. While providing positive evidence for the hypnotic preparation for childbirth, the study was limited to adolescent women and should be followed-up by studies on a wider range of pregnant women in larger numbers.

HYPNO-PSYCHOTHERAPY

In a qualitative study by Taylor and Ingleton (2003), the effects of a combined hypno-psychotherapy programme were evaluated for cancer patients undergoing chemotherapy (see Ch. 11). Eight patients who had completed the programme were selected to take part in the study and semi-structured interviews were conducted an average of 7 months post-intervention. On analysing the interview transcripts, a number of themes were identified. The holding of negative assumptions of hypnosis was observed in participants prior to treatment which suggests that educating the public on the nature of hypnotherapy may still be necessary so they may seek help on an informed basis. Patients appreciated the individualized style of the therapy and felt empowered to take control of their lives after having felt that they had lost this through their cancer journey. Some continued to use the tools that they had learnt in other areas of their lives, underlining the versatility of the treatment. Subjects were purposefully selected for the study so a level of bias may exist while a wider demographical range may also have been useful. An important finding was that healthcare professionals were reticent in referring patients to the scheme. Whether this was through overlooking the psychological needs of patients or whether they had negative preconceptions surrounding hypnotherapy remains unclear but would be the subject of an interesting investigation.

Bryant et al (2005) endeavoured to evaluate the effect of combining hypnosis with cognitive-behavioural therapy (CBT) in the management of acute stress disorder by conducting a well-designed RCT. Participants were randomly allocated to a group receiving supportive counselling, CBT or CBT and hypnosis, while equivalence between groups was sought, based on initial presentation. The CBT-hypnosis group followed the same protocol as the CBT group, apart from being exposed to trance induction and suggestions around an increased involvement and heightened experience during the process. It was noted that fewer participants in the CBT-hypnosis group had re-experienced symptoms of post-traumatic stress disorder at the end of the treatment when compared with those in the CBT group. Both groups were equivalent at 6-month follow-up, however this still produced better results than supportive counselling. Although the results of this study may provide a justification for integrating hypnosis with psychotherapy in acute stress disorder, the authors suggest that the scope of therapeutic gain may have been limited in the way they employed hypnotic techniques. Further research revising how to integrate the two therapies is recommended.

DEMENTIA

Emotionally taxing for all carers involved, Duff and Nightingale (2007) conducted a pilot RCT to investigate if hypnotherapy can improve psychological QOL in people living with dementia. Three groups of six care home residents received either 36 × 1-hour sessions of hypnotherapy, attended 36 × 1-hour discussion groups or received standard care. Quality of life was rated using a questionnaire devised for the study, containing a 7-point Likert scale measuring areas of concentration, relaxation, motivation, activities of daily living, immediate memory, memory for significant events and socialization. Although the questionnaire has not been previously validated, it was based on prior evidence. The nursing staff working within the care homes assessed the ratings through observation. The results show that the average QOL, combining all scores, was higher in the hypnotherapy group during and after the intervention period and that this effect was maintained at a 12-month follow up. Although the assessment by the nursing staff may introduce a study bias, pragmatically it may have been the best way of data capture given the ever-changing nature of dementia. If possible, however, it would be useful to gain perspectives from the individuals. There are, however, ethical concerns in this area. Participants must be able to consent to each treatment but also to the entire project. In this study, care was taken to assess whether or not the participants had the capacity to consent to treatment and to the study, following the relevant legislation. This adherence to legal and ethical guidance should be replicated in any future studies. Given the distressing nature of dementia for patients, their families and carers it is an important area of potential research to focus on, especially given current social trends toward an increasingly ageing population.

HEALTHY HYPNOSIS

In an interesting study, Van de Vusse et al (2006) conducted a prospective study of how hypnosis affected a group of 30 healthy women. For this within-subjects quasi-experimental trial, the participants listened to a 30-minute recorded hypnotherapy session while attached to continuous electro-cardiography. They completed a Profile of Mood States (POMS) questionnaire before and after the session. Results showed a significant reduction in heart rate, respiratory rate and tension-anxiety score from the POMS questionnaire. A greater heart rate variability during hypnosis was observed which the authors suggest indicates better functioning of the parasympathetic nervous system. While the study is not of the highest methodological quality, its novelty of investigating the benefits of hypnotherapy on healthy subjects is worth exploring further. It points to a potentially effective health promotion practice but needs to be researched further with a wider cohort of the population taking part in a well-controlled trial.

PAIN

Although touched upon within the included research into hypnosis during medical procedures, the topic area of pain is vast, as is the scope of its application. It has also been widely studied and so a review by Patterson and Jenson (2003) has been included to reflect this. A literature review occupies the space between the RCT and the systematic review within the hierarchy of evidence. It reviews the literature on a given topic, which may include RCTs, but it does not follow as strict a protocol as a systematic review would. Summarizing their findings, the authors found a wealth of laboratory studies showing that the level of hypnotic analgesia is associated with suggestibility. So the more suggestible a patient is, the more benefit they will derive from it. A review of the trials into the management of acute pain found that hypnotherapy was shown to be effective in the majority of cases. In some cases, however, it was not shown to produce any difference when compared with the control group. Furthermore, hypnotherapy in comparison with other therapies such as relaxation training or distraction was superior only half of the time. In chronic pain studies, hypnosis was shown to be equivalent to acute pain management when compared with controls, however it was less often shown to outperform other therapies like auto-genic and relaxation training. Many of the studies on chronic pain focused on headaches, with positive results, but more investigation into other causes of chronic pain is recommended. Noted also, is that many people live with chronic pain in the community and, encompassing more biopsychosocial issues than acute pain, it is a more complex subject area. It is important to note that the effect of hypnotic analgesia was not shown, in any study, to be less effective than other methods. Thus, the authors conclude that hyp-notherapy is a useful treatment in the management of both acute and chronic pain. This review is an in-depth one, going into the theoretical debates around hypnoanalgesia, and this complicated subject matter is referred to in many of the chapters in this book.

Patterson and Jenson (2003) surveyed brain-imaging studies on hypnotic analgesia and found that hypnosis moderated brain function during the reduction in perceived pain. More recent studies using positron emission tomography (Faymonville et al 2006) and functional magnetic resonance imaging (Mohr et al 2005, Derbyshire et al 2009) support these findings on hypnotically modified neural activity. The researchers concur that areas of the limbic system, like the cingulate cortex, seem to be involved in the anal-gesic effect. The variety of studies into hypnotherapy demonstrates that the research being conducted is building the evidence base showing that hypnotherapy works but also how it works.

RECOMMENDATIONS FOR FUTURE RESEARCH

- Multidimensional chronic pain studies with people living in the community
- Investigate the benefits of hypnotherapy as a health promotion activity
- RCTs of higher internal validity in the management of IBS
- Trials with more equivalence between groups for suggestibility
- An assessment of how well hypnotherapy may integrate with other interventions
- Surveys on attitudes toward hypnotherapy within the healthcare community
- Evaluate the preoperative application of hypnotherapy to postoperative recovery
- Cost-effectiveness analyses into the use of hypnotherapy within medical settings
- Utilizing mixed-methods approach advocated by recent discussions within the research community
- Further investigations into the benefits that older people may draw from hypnotherapeutic interventions.

SUMMARY

This chapter comprises a brief introduction into concepts important in the researching of hypnotherapy as a viable tool within healthcare. It may appear daunting to some but it is only the application of a learned process.

Countless points of reference and advice are easily found when sought and experienced researchers are often happy to assist those that are dipping their toe in the water. The studies included in this chapter are not definitive within the subject, further exploration of the research is always recommended. An awareness of the growing base of evidence should enable a practicing hypnotherapist to feel confident about their practice and of the difference that they can make in others. The findings of hypnotherapy research are important to therapists, healthcare professionals and to the consumers and commissioners of health services. It is hoped that therapists and healthcare professionals alike can embrace a research approach to practice, and use its light to inform and improve patient care and choices. As CAM research booms, becoming its own discipline, the findings generated can underline the healing effects that can be produced from the eloquently simple use of voice, rhythm and the weaving of words.

REFERENCES

Block, K.I., Burns, B., Cohen, A.J., et al., 2004. Point-counterpoint: using clinical trials for the evaluation of integrative cancer therapies. Integr. Cancer Ther. 3 (1), 66–81.

Broom, A., Adams, J., 2007. Current issues and future directions in complementary and alternative medicine research. Complement. Ther. Med. 15 (3), 217–220.

Bryant, R., Moulds, M., Guthrie, R., et al., 2005. The additive effect of hypnosis and cognitive-behavioural therapy in treating acute stress disorder. J. Consult. Clin. Psychol. 73 (2), 334–340.

Derbyshire, S.W., Whalley, M.G., Oakley, D.A., 2009. Fibromyalgia pain and its modulation by hypnotic and non-hypnotic suggestion: an fMRI analysis. Eur. J. Pain 13 (5), 542–550.

DoH, 2005. The research governance framework for health and social care, second ed. Department of Health, London.

Duff, S., Nightingale, D., 2007. Alternative approaches to supporting individuals with dementia: enhancing quality of life with hypnosis. Alzheimer's Care Today 8 (4), 321–331.

Faymonville, M., Boly, M., Laureys, S., 2006. Functional neuroanatomy of the hypnotic state. J. Physiol. (Paris) 99 (4–6), 463–469.

Gholamrezaei, A., Emami, M.H., 2008. How to put hypnosis into a placebo pill? Complement. Ther. Med. 16, 52–54.

Gonsalkorale, W.M., Houghton, L.A., Whorwell, P.J., 2002. Hypnotherapy in irritable bowel syndrome: a large-scale audit of a clinical service with examination of factors influencing responsiveness. Am. J. Gastroenterol. 97 (4), 954–961.

House of Lords Select Committee on Science and Technology – Sixth Report, 2000. Complementary and alternative medicine. The Stationery Office, London.

Lang, E.V., Benotsch, E.G., Fick, L.J., et al., 2000. Adjunctive non-pharmacological analgesia for invasive medical procedures: a randomised trial. Lancet 355 (9214), 1486–1490.

Lang, E.V., Berbaum, K.S., Pauker, S.G., et al., 2008. Beneficial effects of hypnosis and adverse effects of empathic attention during percutaneous tumour treatment: when being nice does not suffice. J. Vasc. Interv. Radiol. 19 (6), 897–905.

Lewith, G., 2003. Misconceptions about research in complementary medicine. In: Vickers, A. (Ed.), Examining complementary medicine. Stanley Thomas, Cheltenham.

Liossi, C., White, P., Hatire, P., 2006. Randomised clinical trial of local anaesthetic versus a combination of local anaesthetic with self-hypnosis in the management of paediatric procedure-related pain. Health Psychol. 25 (3), 307–315.

Martin, A.A., Schauble, P.G., Rai, S.H., et al., 2001. Effects of hypnosis on the labour processes and birth outcomes of pregnant adolescents. J. Fam. Pract. 50, 441–443.

Mohr, C., Binkofski, S., Erdmann, C., et al., 2005. The anterior cingulate cortex contains distinct areas dissociating external from self-administered painful stimulation: a parametric fMRI study. Pain 114 (3), 347–357.

Ozturk, A., 2006. Using hypnosis in a case of cholecystectomy, a case report. Eur. J. Pain 10 (1), S226.

Patterson, D.R., Jensen, M., 2003. Hypnosis and clinical pain control. Psychol. Bull. 129 (4), 495–521.

Reynolds, S., 2000. The anatomy of evidence-based practice: principles and methods. In: Trinder, L., Reynolds, S. (Eds.), Evidence-based practice: a critical appraisal. Blackwell Science, Oxford.

Saadat, H., Drummond-Lewis, J., Maranets, I., et al., 2006. Hypnosis reduces preoperative anxiety in adult patients. Anesth. Analg. 102 (5), 1394–1396.

Sackett, D.L., Straus, S., Richardson, W.S., et al., 2000. Evidence-based Medicine: How to practice and teach EBM, second ed. Churchill Livingstone, Edinburgh.

Seedhouse, D., 1998. Ethics: the heart of healthcare, second ed. Wiley & Sons, Chichester.

Taylor, E.E., Ingleton, C., 2003. Hypnotherapy and cognitive-behavioural therapy in cancer care: the patients' view. Eur. J. Cancer Care (Engl) 12 (2), 137–142.

Tonelli, M.R., Callahan, T.C., 2003. Why alternative medicine cannot be evidence-based. Acad. Med. 76 (12), 1213–1220.

Van de Vusse, L., Berner, M., White-Winters, J.M., 2006. A prospective pre-post comparison of physiologic and psychologic variables in child-bearing aged women experiencing hypnosis. J. Midwifery Womens Health 51 (5), 389.

Verhoef, M.J., Lewith, G., Ritenbaugh, C., et al., 2005. Complementary and alternative medicine whole systems research: beyond identification of inadequacies of the RCT. Complement. Ther. Med. 13, 206–212.

Vincent, C., Furnham, A., 1998. Complementary medicine: a research perspective. Wiley, London.

Wilson, S., Maddison, T., Roberts, L., et al., 2006. Systematic review: the effectiveness of hypnotherapy in the management of irritable bowel syndrome. Aliment. Pharmacol. Ther. 24 (5), 769–780.

FURTHER READING

Ernst, E., 2007. Understanding research in complementary and alternative medicine. EMS, London.

Lewith, G.T., Jones, W.B., Walach, H., 2001. Clinical research in complementary therapies: principles, problems and solutions. Churchill Livingstone, London.

Long, T., Johnson, M., 2006. Research ethics in the real world. Issues and solutions for health and social care. Churchill Livingstone, Edinburgh.

Polgar, S., Thomas, S.A., 2000. Introduction to research in the health sciences, fourth ed. Churchill Livingstone, London.

USEFUL RESOURCES

Complementary Therapy and Smoking Cessation Services, Rehabilitation Unit, The Christie NHS Foundation Trust, Wilmslow Road, Manchester M20 4BX, UK. Website: www.christie.nhs.uk/patients/rehab/comp/default.aspx.

London College of Clinical Hypnosis, 27 Gloucester Place, London W1U 8HU, UK. Website: www.lcch.co.uk.

Medical School Hypnosis Association, Department of Health and Human Sciences, London Metropolitan University, 166–220 Holloway Road, London N7 8DB, UK. Website: www.msha.org.uk.

Working with the therapeutic relationship

Anne Cawthorn • Bernadette Shepherd

CHAPTER CONTENTS

CHAPTER OUTLINE

This chapter reviews the significance of the therapeutic relationship within hypnotherapy. Key issues are raised with regard to the role of positive expectations in therapeutic change, with an emphasis on the ways that therapists, who use hypnosis, can take advantage of what may be strong,

© 2010 Elsevier Ltd.
DOI: 10.1016/B978-0-7020-3082-6.00007-1

positive effects for their patients. Case studies are included to illustrate the 'clinical feel' alongside theoretical ideas. The literature relating to the therapeutic relationship is explored, while introducing an assessment model in addition to a model which guides hypnotherapy practice.

KEY WORDS

Therapeutic
Relationship
DIRECT (Model 1)
I CHOOSE (Model 2)
Empathy
Positive expectancy

INTRODUCTION

The relationship between patient and therapist is unique. A therapeutic relationship has in its very existence a commitment to the well-being of one person, the patient. Moursand and Erskine (2003) suggest that the business of establishing and maintaining a therapeutic relationship requires a delicate balance, involved but not demanding, vulnerable but not weak, willing to share self-awareness but not imposing that self-awareness onto the patient. In relationship hypnotherapy, the therapist enters consciously into the relationship with the patient and creates a safe space in which the relationship itself supports and encourages change.

The late Milton H. Erickson is renowned as a master hypnotist and as a therapist without par. Lynn and Hallquist (2004) argue that Eriksson's clinical proficiency was as attributable to his ability to forge strong therapeutic relationships as to his use of particular hypnotic techniques. Erikson's utilization approach enabled him to gain the cooperation and trust of many of his clients and to establish a strong therapeutic alliance. This in turn enhanced rapport, which is essential for optimizing hypnotic responsiveness (Lynn & Hallquist 2004). Indeed, Erickson was so successful as a therapist due to many of his creative techniques being effective in establishing a strong working alliance. Nuttall (2002) describes the working alliance as the understanding that patient and therapist have in order to cooperate in the therapeutic process. It is that element of the relationship, established outside all others, that enables two individuals to work together.

Factors that influence positive hypnotherapy outcome can be divided into two main areas: common factors and positive expectancy effects.

COMMON FACTORS

Common factors such as empathy, warmth and the therapeutic relationship have been shown to correlate more highly with patient outcome than specialized treatment interventions. The common factors most frequently studied have been person-centred facilitative conditions (empathy, warmth, congruence) and the therapeutic alliance (Lambert & Barley 2001). Decades of research indicate the provision of therapy, including hypnotherapy, is an interpersonal process in which a main curative component is the nature of the therapeutic relationship (Patterson 1985, Bird 1993, Lambert & Barley 2001). Patients often attribute their positive therapy outcome to the personal attributes of their therapist (Lazarus 1971, Bird 1993, Safran 1993, Howe 1999). Patients who felt their therapy was successful described their therapist as warm, attentive, interested, understanding and respectful (Howe 1999, Lambert & Barley 2001). Similarly, in a large comprehensive review of over 2000 studies since 1950, Orlinsky et al (1994) identified several therapist variables and behaviours which have consistently been shown to have a positive impact on treatment outcome. Key factors such as therapist credibility, skill, empathic understanding and affirmation of the patient's problems, and directing the patient's attention to the affective experience, were related to successful treatment.

POSITIVE EXPECTANCY EFFECTS

The importance of positive expectancy (the patient's beliefs, motivations and attitudes) cannot be emphasized enough. Kirsch (1990), based on clear empirical evidence, suggests that a person's positive expectancy that he or she is likely to produce a given behaviour (e.g. positive outcomes in hypnotherapy) is the single best predictor of that behaviour. Spanos and Coe (1992) report that the more the patient's expectations are in agreement with the therapist's, the more likely it is that they will be good hypnotic subjects. However, if a patient is unwilling to cooperate, he or she cannot be hypnotized; the potential hypnotic patient must be motivated to enter the relationship. The closer the patient's expectations for their conduct match the requests of the therapist, the more likely they are to be responsive. Spanos and Coe (1992) highlight that coupled with motivational factors are certain abilities that appear to be useful in hypnosis (i.e. concentration and absorbed imagining). In keeping with the concept of expectancy, Barrios (1970) viewed the hypnotic induction as an effective method for establishing confidence and belief in the therapist. In addition, a strong personal relationship should develop wherein the therapists' words should be more effective in bringing about constructive change.

Horvarth and Symonds (1991: 366), reporting on a meta analysis of 90 independent clinical investigations, conclude that: 'It is likely that a little over half of the beneficial effects of psychotherapy, for example, accounted for in previous meta-analysis, are linked to the quality of the therapeutic alliance'. Research undertaken by Lambert and Okiishi (1997) estimated that only 15% of change can be attributed to specific techniques (with some exceptions); the other 85% of a client's improvement can be attributed to factors such as the therapeutic relationship. Horvarth and Bedi's (2002) review on the literature on the therapeutic alliance concludes that establishing a strong alliance is crucial to its ultimate success. Horvarth and Bedi (2002) go on to discuss a number of therapist variables that appear to be related to an effective therapeutic alliance, included are: communication skills, experience and training, personality and intrapersonal process, and collaboration with the client. There are things identified that can be specified about creating and utilizing a good therapeutic relationship and many of these things can be taught directly.

UTILIZATION APPROACH

Considerable evidence indicates that rapport is also important, especially in optimizing hypnotic responsiveness (Lynn & Hallquist 2004). Erickson's utilization approach enabled him to gain the cooperation and trust of many of his clients and to establish a rapid and strong therapeutic alliance (Hayley 1973). In this respect, the therapist utilizes the patient's ongoing behaviour, perceptions, and attitudes in facilitating therapeutic change. Patients are not asked to conform to the therapist's mode of interaction; rather, their behaviour is accepted and utilized in the treatment process. This utilization process would include direct and indirect suggestions. Erickson et al (1976) noted that indirect suggestion permits the patient's individuality, previous life experience and unique potential to become manifest. Hammond (1984) noted that Erickson relied heavily on indirect suggestion in the latter part of his career. He observed that indirection allowed him to show respect for his patients by not directly challenging them to do what the conscious mind, for whatever reason, would not do. Lankton and Lankton (1983) indicated that indirection is the basis for the therapeutic use of metaphors, and stories, because they allow patients to make meaning relevant for them and to explore their potential to facilitate new responses.

Erickson created a strong therapeutic alliance in the way he displayed respect for his client's beliefs. He did not impose his position and perspective on the client; rather he paid close attention to the client's reality. He was a master of rapport building technique, using what the client said or did as a starting place and built on it to establish and preserve positive treatment expectancies and rapport. Erickson capitalized on the positive expectations of his clients regarding hypnosis. Erickson often defined his work with clients as 'hypnotic' in nature, whether or not he used a formal induction, or whether his clients discussed their experiences in terms of trance or 'hypnosis'. There is substantial research support for the idea that simply labelling procedures as 'hypnotic' can enhance treatment outcomes (Kirsch 1997).

A good therapeutic relationship increases the power expectancy of a hypnotic intervention and the client's willingness to be affected by it, and we agree with Gehrie (1999: 87) that: 'The relationship is not the treatment but the relationship makes the treatment possible if it is properly managed'.

DEVELOPING THE HYPNOTHERAPEUTIC RELATIONSHIP

Building and developing a therapeutic relationship based on important skills of inquiry, attunement and involvement allows for hypnotherapy to be integrated and applied therapeutically to the patient and not as a problem-solving technique. This approach involves conveying to the patient a sense of acceptance; a feeling that the patient genuinely feels heard and understood. A strong therapeutic alliance with a foundation of empathy and therapist presence provides the framework that allows in-depth exploration to occur.

THE TRAVELLING COMPANION

Ebell (2008) regards the therapeutic alliance as a joint venture, one in which the therapist and patient join in a cooperative search for potential changes. The patient examines his or her resources, as well as relevant obstacles and conflicts. Short et al (2005) reported how Erickson clearly placed 'hypnotherapy' as an adjunct to other concepts. His emphasis was on the inner resources of the patient and not the actions of the therapist. He maintained that people have more potential and resources than they realize, and hypnosis has the ability to evoke the hidden potential of the client.

The term 'travelling companion' has been voiced by Ebell (2008) as the position that a therapist can take when working with patients who are chronically ill. The patient and therapist embark as travelling companions on a journey together through entirely uncharted territories. The onset of the journey involves paying close attention to the patient's explanation of his or her subjective experience with suffering. Ebell (2008) goes on to suggest that one of the most potent ways to develop the relationship alliance, is to use the patient's language and language pattern. In the practice of hypnosis, encouraging patients to re-examine their experiences and explanations can, in itself, prove instrumental in the promotion of change (Ebell 2008).

BUILDING THE THERAPEUTIC ALLIANCE

Establishing a strong therapeutic alliance in the early stages of hypnotherapy is crucial to its ultimate success. Lynn and Hallquist (2004) describe how Erickson, in his initial contact with patients, would acknowledge to them that there were some things that they might not want to share, and he encouraged them to withhold such information. However, as the patients disclosed one thing after another, they would begin to withhold less and less and to ultimately tell Erickson what they had set out not to mention (Hayley 1985). This rapport-building technique illustrates Erickson's skills in encouraging the client's narrative and in developing a therapeutic alliance.

EMPATHY

Key to the building of a therapeutic alliance is empathy. The skill of empathic understanding is the foundation store for the hypnotherapy technique that the therapist may use. The most basic ingredient in the empathic process is attending: listening to what the patient says, noticing what they do, and being fully and actively involved in the process. In our attempt to understand the patient, we must take care not to make the patient some 'out there' thing, totally separate and distinct from ourselves (Moursand & Erskine 2003). We too are part of the equation; our understanding of the patient is impacted by our own history and expectations. Tansy and Burke (1989) suggest we listen from within; our own responses are the guide we use to interpret and give meaning to what the patient says and does. As Bascal (1997: 670) puts it, 'Empathy effectively constitutes a reading of the analyst's own affects and ... when we 'emphasize' we are always interpreting the effect of our subjectivity of what the patient feels, believes, or does'.

Empathy in this context underpins Eriksonian approaches, or, synonymously, utilization approaches (Erickson et al 1976). Hypnosis in this view is a result of a focused and meaningful reaction between therapist and patient. The therapist to be successful must be responsive to the needs of the patient and tailor his or her approach to those needs, if the patient is going to be at all responsive to the possibilities of change. A patient's behaviour and feelings are fed back to him or her verbally/non-verbally, thereby creating a sense in the patient of being understood, which is the essence of rapport (Yapko 2003). Hypnosis is considered a natural outcome of a relationship where each participant is responsive to the sensitive following and leading of the other. Yapko (2003) encourages the therapist to actively refrain from the undesirable approach of imposing their beliefs and values on to their patient. The interactional view emphasizes responsiveness and respect for the patient, which is ideal in the hypnotherapeutic context. Lynn and Hallquist (2004: 64) go as far as to suggest that a skilled practitioner of hypnosis lacking familiarity with Erikson's approach to hypnosis is akin to a physicist lacking familiarity with quantum mechanics.

When exploring the practice of hypnosis, it is as a tool and as such it should not stand alone. Therapists, therefore, incorporating hypnotherapy into their practice, should not solely rely on their skill and confidence in mastering the techniques, but also on the establishment of a strong therapeutic alliance. This view is supported by others from the field of hypnotherapy. Yapko (1992) suggests that many clinicians today adopt the view that clinical hypnosis is not a therapy in its own right, but merely a vehicle or tool for delivering information, increasing client responsiveness and to facilitate experiential work with clients. More recently, the APA's Division of Psychological Hypnosis (1999) (Yapko 2001) also stated that hypnosis is not a therapy but a procedure to facilitate therapy. They go on to say that it is not a treatment in itself because the training in hypnosis is not sufficient for the conduct of therapy.

When reflecting on the developing relationship within hypnotherapy, Yapko (2001) urges us to be aware of the following important distinction; suggesting that the practitioner should consider whether they are actually 'doing hypnosis' vs 'being hypnotic.' He goes on to say that someone who reads a script to a client may be doing hypnosis, whereas he suggests that being hypnotic is:

> Engaging purposefully with people, accepting the responsibility for being an agent of influence and change, and striving to use the capacity for influence intelligently and sensitively.

Yapko (2001: 26)

ASSESSMENT MODEL

Good assessment skills are the key to any therapeutic relationship as it allows the therapist to get to know the person and explore their concerns and to negotiate how to work using hypnotherapy techniques. The DIRECT/Negotiation Model is a framework to elicit and manage clients' concerns. The model was initially developed as an assessment tool to elicit sexual concerns (Cawthorn & Fielding 2006). (A full description of the model can be found at: www://learnzone.macmillan.org.uk.) It has at its core the Maguire assessment model, which was originally developed to improve

> **BOX 5.1 The DIRECT/Negotiation Model: A 6-stage approach to assessment**
>
> 1. **D**evelop the relationship/negotiate before moving on
> 2. **I**nvite the person to tell you about themselves and inquire how any concerns they have impact on them as an individual/negotiate
> 3. **R**eflect back your willingness to hear their concerns/negotiate
> 4. **E**licit and **E**xplore their concerns/negotiate
> 5. **C**ommunicate your understanding of their problem and negotiate how these might be resolved
> 6. **T**reatment/therapy can be negotiated and suggestions made as to how hypnotherapy techniques can help in resolving their concerns.

healthcare professionals' skills in assessing and communicating with cancer patients and has been adopted and taught both in the UK and worldwide (Parle et al 1997).

The DIRECT/Negotiation Model (Box 5.1) utilizes a staged approach to assessment allowing the therapist and patient to proceed at a mutually agreed level. It is particularly useful when negotiating whether the client wishes to work with particularly sensitive areas. Negotiation is used to elicit what the patient is comfortable working with. It is used throughout the assessment, enabling the therapist to proceed at the patient's pace. This can relate to either the depth of communication they are comfortable with, or when negotiating which hypnotherapy approaches they are happy to engage in.

DEVELOP THE RELATIONSHIP

Developing a good relationship with the client is the first step in any assessment process. It entails the therapist 'getting into step with them' and 'learning their dance'. 'The therapist's skill is in inviting them on to the dance floor, guiding and showing them that they can trust in the relationship' (Cawthorn 2006: 73).

Before commencing, ensure that the following three core components are present:

- Privacy: this helps both the client and therapist feel comfortable
- Permission: is a 2-way process:
  - Permission needs to be given by the *therapist* that they are okay listening to the person's concerns. This requires them to develop a high level of self-awareness, learning to be comfortable with any issues, especially the more sensitive ones such as sexuality, abuse, existential issues relating to mortality and dying (see Chs 9 and 14)
  - Permission needs to be gained from the *patient* as to whether they are comfortable sharing some of their more intimate concerns with you
- Potency: requires awareness by the therapist as to their level of competency and to know when to refer on or seek extra supervision.

The following steps can enhance the process of developing the relationship.

Develop a conversational approach

Hobson (1985) describes this as a way of communicating, which entails relating 'person to person'. Be aware of the client's non-verbal cues and your own in response. Make sure that your non-verbal cues are conveying that you are open and comfortable discussing their concerns. Remember that a wealth of information can be obtained just from observing the person's body language and you can observe whether what they are saying matches up with what you are observing from their body language. Develop rapport by using their language. Rapport is 'the natural process of matching and being in alignment with another person' (Andreas & Faulkner 1996: 334). By reflecting back the words people offer you in an empathic way, this helps to begin the process of developing rapport. Mirroring or matching the person's body language also gives out subtle messages, thereby increasing rapport.

Listen to and inquire about the metaphors people use to describe their experiences

A metaphor is an indirect figure of speech which implies a comparison of something (O'Connor 2001). It is something which is used in place of another and as such, we may think we understand what the metaphor is implying, but to truly know, we need to inquire what the person means by its use. Common metaphors used by people relate to: the journey, a roller coaster ride, martial or fighting metaphors or conversely healing ones. A common metaphor used by patients to describe the experience surrounding their illness and treatment relates to the fairground. Listening to people use this metaphor evokes in the therapist their own personal images of the fairground. However, when inquiring with the client what their understanding of this is, a very different image often arises (see Box 5.2, Case study 1).

INVITE THE PERSON TO TELL YOU ABOUT THEMSELVES AND INQUIRE HOW THEIR EXPERIENCES HAVE IMPACTED ON THEM

It is very empowering to be invited by an interested person to talk about yourself. The therapist might ask the patient: 'tell me something about yourself as an individual' or inquire 'how are you coping with the situation you

---

BOX 5.2 Case study 1

Susan, a 37-year-old lady with breast cancer likened all her treatments, including surgery, chemotherapy and radiotherapy, as similar to being at the fairground. She recalled that 'each treatment was like being put on a different ride at the fair, and each time I was taken off one ride, I would be put on to another, equally terrifying ride, which I had no control over!'

This particular metaphor gave a wealth of information about Susan's experience and offered material to work with using hypnotherapy techniques. The aim of working was to change the metaphor into a much more positive one which Susan was able to cope with. In addition, we worked together on how Susan could gain control in what felt an 'out of control' situation by accessing and stacking a number of positive anchors from her past.

find yourself in?' Additionally, the therapist might ask 'what helps you to cope/doesn't help?' By allowing patients an opportunity to tell their narrative, this in turn gives the therapist a window into their conscious world. Later, when moving on to utilize hypnotherapy techniques we are then offered a privileged view into the world of their unconscious. By having the former information, the therapist and the patient are in the enlightened position to be able to compare the two for similarities or differences.

Normalizing is an important skill when used appropriately. Often, people assume they are the only ones having a difficult reaction to the situation they are in. A useful way of helping people is by using phrases that normalize the subject without minimizing it. Examples might be:

It is not uncommon to have difficulty sleeping or vivid dreams following a difficult experience and I wonder if this has been the same for you?

Some people have a sense of loss similar to a bereavement following an amputation, heart attack, stroke ... and I was wondering if this had happened to you.

If a patient says 'yes', negotiate whether they want to discuss their concerns, as some may acknowledge your inquiry, but not necessarily want to proceed to exploring their concerns.

REFLECT BACK YOUR WILLINGNESS TO HEAR THEIR CONCERNS

If the patient wants to discuss their problems, this is the time to let them know that you are willing to hear their concerns. This can be done by reflecting back the information which they have already given you.

If the person does not want to explore them further at this time (it may be too soon), leave the door open for further discussion in the future. You will still have validated the individual's concerns and given them permission to share now or later. This may also help the patient to begin clarifying their concerns, prior to articulating them. Never underestimate how important it is to be listened to and to have someone communicate back their understanding of what they have heard to you.

COMMUNICATE

Communicate with the patient as to your understanding of their concerns, while checking out whether your understanding matches theirs. It allows you the opportunity to negotiate how you will work together in a way that would best suit them.

Negotiate with the patient whether they would like hypnotherapy for the identified concerns.

THERAPY: INCLUDING HYPNOTHERAPY

This is where you contract to work together using appropriate hypnotherapy techniques. The Hypnotherapy Practice Model I CHOOSE, devised by the authors, gives a framework for hypnotherapy practice which is explained below.

HYPNOTHERAPY PRACTICE MODEL: I CHOOSE

I = INTENTION

Intention is working in a purposeful way with a goal in mind. It involves focussing on the person and includes ownership, having an awareness of the other and self by matching intention. It is not about leading or being overly directive, but working with the other person to reach the desired outcome. Campbell (1984) sees the therapist as being a skilled companion on the patient's journey, while working with respect and reverence. O'Connor (2001: 40) reminds us that when working with someone, we need to develop trust, which he suggests 'is a gift you bestow on another' and without trust, the ability to work together is limited. However, he reminds us that 'trust is a risk and a delicate dance with another person that takes time to manifest' (O'Connor 2001). In order to judge if the person is able to trust us, we need to ask the question 'how strong are they? And how vulnerable are you as the therapist prepared to be?'

C = CONTRACT

All therapy should include a contract which is agreed between the patient and therapist. However, it is even more important with hypnotherapy practice, as the patient needs to be aware they have consented to the use of trance and any hypnotherapy techniques which the therapist has suggested. Hypnotic procedures should be administered only with the patient's consent. Ideally this should avoid being a verbal contract which is loose and open to abuse and misinterpretation. It should be a written contract which includes confidentiality, the patient's right of access to the complaints procedure of the hypnotherapies governing body and informed consent.

Gaining informed consent from the patient provides the therapist with an opportunity to describe the procedures to the patient and to create realistic expectations as to the outcome. The contract is an opportunity for the therapist to create a positive expectation of hypnosis and to clear up misconceptions. Patient anxiety about hypnosis can be reduced by demystifying the procedures, thereby helping the patient to feel more in control. Explaining the procedure of hypnosis in a straightforward relaxed manner to the patient during contract making reduces the likelihood of a negative reaction (Overholser 1988).

H = HEALING

Over the past 20 years, there has been a wealth of literature discussing the concept of healing and it is now much more acceptable to use the term within healthcare. The term healing comes from the Old English 'haelen', to make whole, and perhaps one of the reasons for its acceptance is aligned to the increase in holistic practice. Cunningham (2000) suggests that healing and understanding are closely aligned and the more we try to understand our patients and communicate this understanding to them, this can have a healing effect. Seigal (2001) advises that the doctor is the facilitator of healing, not the healer himself and goes on to suggest that doctors and patients should see each other as joint participants in a healing process to which each brings qualities of mind and heart.

Cunningham (2000) asserts that connection improves healing just as separateness between parts and levels of the person, promotes disease of the body. This would explain how the therapeutic relationship between client and therapist can be healing in itself as it helps people to take control, get connected and begin the process of self-understanding. The use of hypnotherapy allows the patient to get in touch with both the conscious and unconscious, to consult with their 'Inner Healer' in the imagination and to bring about healing from within (Cunningham 2000). When people access the wealth of information which the unconscious holds, they can gain new information about their body and mind which can then be used to bring about healing. The therapist is the privileged facilitator of this.

O = OPENNESS

Openness is an essential ingredient in the therapeutic encounter between the therapist and patient. A hypnotherapist, who is open to all possibilities within the encounter, allows the facilitation of what can be an amazing journey of discovery between themselves and the patient. The opposite of openness is referred to as blocking where people do not feel safe and supported in the moment and are potentially discounting physical and/or psychological aspects of their personalities. Openness can be developed through supervision and a supportive relationship outside of the therapeutic work (Johns 2004). Cunningham (2000) suggests that an information flow from 'mind', 'social level' and 'spiritual', is included in the accounts of healing possibilities.

O = OPTIONS

Options refers to the choices the therapist can offer the client when they are negotiating how they would like to work. If the person has never received hypnotherapy before, or utilized similar techniques such as visualization or relaxation, then time, explaining what is entailed, is time well spent. Experience has often shown that unless there is an urgent need to proceed rapidly (e.g. when people have a phobia which is stopping them having urgent treatment), then time spent developing the relationship, building rapport and experiencing light trance may set the foundations for further therapeutic encounters. As there are usually a number of options which can be utilized to benefit certain problems, the skill of the therapist lies in assessing and negotiating which would best suit the client at this time. It is appropriate to share some options with the client because they are usually the best judge of what would be right for them. Clients are more creative than we often give them credit for and can go to places, during a session, which we had not anticipated during the initial assessment.

S = SAFETY

Safety should always be of great importance in any therapeutic encounter. However, where trance work is involved, safety needs to be paramount.

There are numerous reasons why people may feel unsafe when deciding to engage in hypnotherapy, some of which will be explored further.

It is not unusual for clients to experience some initial apprehension about being a recipient of hypnotherapy. This could originate from witnessing stage hypnosis, and if this is the case, they will need reassurance and information regarding how the approaches differ. Another possibility is that they may have received hypnotherapy in the past which did not meet their needs, or where the practitioner's skills were limited.

In addition, if the therapeutic relationship had not been successfully developed, this could also have influenced their confidence relating to this type of therapy. The most common situation is usually that the client has no experience, or limited knowledge, regarding hypnotherapy. At this point they may not feel unsafe, just unsure, and with proper information this could be resolved.

Loss of control is another area about which clients openly express their nervousness when considering receiving hypnotherapy. Again, information about the nature of trance should help to reassure the person as well as giving them the opportunity to have any questions answered, in a way that demystifies hypnotherapy. A good therapist can allay these fears by taking time to assess the person and explain what is involved in using hypnotherapy techniques. It is always useful to remind people that trance is an everyday phenomenon similar to daydreaming, meditation or absorption in a book and as such, it remains relatively safe because people are able to focus their attention back to normal day activities whenever they wish (Griffin & Tyrell 2003, Heap & Aravind 2002).

Another safety issue relates to the environment where the session takes place. As therapists, we get used to our surroundings and the associated noises. However, we need to be mindful that for the client this may not be the case. Wherever possible the same room should be used each time. Before inducing trance, the client needs to be in a comfortable position, and free from interruptions and extraneous noises. This is possibly easier to achieve in private practice, than in healthcare settings. Even with the best plans, sessions occasionally can be interrupted and unexpected external noises impact on the session.

It is important therefore that the therapist negotiates with the clients to ignore any noises they may hear, as it is the therapist's responsibility to keep them safe. A useful suggestion goes something like 'with every sound that you hear you will become more and more relaxed' or 'every sound that you hear allows you to let go of any stress and tension so you become more and more relaxed'. These statements or similar ones can be repeated again if noises occur or if a noise persists. Personal experience has shown that if the therapist remains calm and grounded in relation to unexpected noises, the client will either fail to notice, or not be affected by the noise.

This is not surprising when looking at the definition of trance. Heap and Aravind (2002: 25) suggest that in trance 'the person's attention is focused away from his or her surroundings and absorbed by inner experiences such as feelings, cognitions and imagery'; they go on to say that in this focused state of attention, the wider environmental stimuli are ignored. Case study 2 (Box 5.3) illustrates this process.

BOX 5.3 Case study 2

Betty was a 47-year-old woman who had been receiving psychotherapy for about 3 months and about to experience her first contracted session using hypnotherapy techniques. I had prepared Betty for the session and discussed what trance entailed. The room should have been free from noise and I noted that construction work was due to start the following week. Betty easily went into a deep trance and we started working together. Just at that moment, a digger started underneath the window, went on to dig a trench and then boarded up the window plunging us into complete darkness. I decided to put the light on and check how Betty was coping. She was oblivious to the noise and what was happening, so we continued with what was a very powerful session. I was taping the session and when I played it back I sounded like 'Kate Adie reporting from a war zone!'

When I evaluated the session with Betty, including the noise, she said that it was fine as she had total trust in me. The lesson being that if we stay grounded and stay focussed the client will follow.

E = ENGAGE

Engaging in hypnotherapy is a 2-way process requiring both the client and the therapist to be connected. One way to check out how connected you are with the person is to look at the polar opposite, by exploring the concept of separateness.

Three important skills which help to facilitate this process are the use of: inquiry, attunement and involvement. Erskine et al (1999) describe this as going beyond empathy to developing a contact form of therapy with the relationship at the core.

One way of describing the situation where the therapist is attuned to the patient on every level including their thoughts, feelings, behaviours and bodily sensations of the patient and themselves, could be called advanced attunement. This is achieved through a 2-way flow of information. Shaw (2004) refers to this concept as embodiment and the results of his phenomenological study with psychotherapists found it to be a common factor. Other authors have described it as embodied countertransference and Samuels (1993: 33) openly acknowledges that 'the analyst's bodily reactions are an important part of the picture. The body is an organ of information'. Rowan (1998) takes Samuels' notion of embodied transference even further, bringing in the idea of linking, which describes a special type of empathy.

When reflecting on personal hypnotherapy practice there have been many times when the connection between the author as the therapist, and the patient, has had a heightened 2-way flow of information, which has enhanced the therapeutic process. Examples of this would be experiencing the same imagery as the patient while they were in their special place during trance. Reflecting on the session, inquiring what the patient saw, it has often been identical to the one imagined they were sensing. Sometimes it relates to their need for a companion on their journey and they can be asked whether they would like to choose one. On other occasions, there is a strong link to

> **BOX 5.4 Case study 3**
>
> Margaret, a 41-year-old lady was having hypnotherapy to help her cope with her chemotherapy. On one session, we were working to make the veins in her right arm more amenable to venopuncture. The permissive approach allowed her to choose the correct temperature for her arm (heat usually facilitates this). At one point in the session, my right arm went very cold, which, on inquiry mirrored her own. On the following session we used a trauma cure to wipe out the memories of a difficult experience during a hospital stay. At one point I became aware of an overwhelming heat which lasted for a period of time during the session. On evaluating the session with Margaret, she recalled that she had been very hot and breathless in part of the traumatic memory she was attempting to wipe.

the temperature which the patient is experiencing during hypnotherapy. This is evident in Case study 3, Box 5.4, when working with a patient who was receiving intravenous chemotherapy.

IMPLICATIONS FOR PROFESSIONAL SUPPORT AND DEVELOPMENT

As hypnotherapy becomes more recognized as a profession, there is greater need for clinical and academic accountability. In the training of hypnotherapists, psychotherapists and counsellors, clinical supervision is now generally accepted as a statutory requirement. Support and guidance are essential underpinnings to therapists working with patients, which is especially important with vulnerable people. There is a need for therapists to be aware of personal thoughts and feelings and how they might influence exchanges between patient and therapist. Jones (1997) indicates that curiosity and fears, within the safe context of clinical supervision, can be used to explore some of the more difficult situations such as working with patients with serious illness or the terminally ill. Therapists' self-awareness and their ability to look at their own issues play a vital role in work of this nature. Any difficulties with the therapeutic relationship should be taken to clinical supervision and in some cases, personal therapy. Within the safe environment of clinical supervision, supervisors and supervisees can examine their own interpersonal processes and can take that learning back into their work with patients.

Given also the importance of facilitative conditions and the therapeutic relationship, training in relationship skills is crucial for therapists. Emphasis should be based on how best to establish and maintain a strong relationship with their patients. Such training should address the therapeutic context, e.g. safe environment, respect for the patient, empathic listening, responding to the patient's concerns.

In this chapter, the authors have emphasized the importance of the therapeutic relationship and suggested that hypnosis is an adjunct to the treatment process, not a treatment in itself. Research demonstrates a good predictor of the hypno-psychotherapy outcome is the therapeutic relationship. With this in mind, therapists have a responsibility to ensure familiarity with up-to-date, relevant research, exploring the factors enhancing the therapeutic relationship, while staying abreast of current and new techniques within the field.

CONCLUSION

This chapter has reviewed both theoretically and empirically the importance of establishing a therapeutic relationship of trust and acceptance with patients. The importance of building a good rapport and working with the role of positive expectations in therapeutic change cannot be over emphasized if the patient is going to engage in the process of hypnosis. Therapists should be alert to the critical role that expectations play in their practice. Clinical case studies have been included in order to illustrate the clinical picture along with the theoretical ideas. In addition an assessment model and hypnotherapy practice model have been explored as frameworks for practice. Emphasizing relationship and other common factors in practice and research is likely to enhance patient outcome far more than solely focusing on the specific technique of hypnosis.

Utilizing hypnosis techniques requires the therapist to build a strong therapeutic alliance with the patient. Hypnosis works within a strong therapeutic relationship by drawing on the intrinsic resources of the patient. Within this process, the patient acts as participant and decision-maker of their progress. All the information to achieve symptom relief or healing is carried within the patients themselves (Ebell 2008).

REFERENCES

Andreas, S., Faulkner, C., 1996. NLP the new technology of achievement. WS Bookwell, Finland.

Barrios, A., 1970. Hypnotherapy: a reappraisal. Psychotherapy Theory Research and Practice 21, 2–7.

Bascal, H.A., 1997. The analyst's subjectivity – how it can illuminate the analysand's experience. Commentary on Susan H. Sand's paper. Psychoanalytic Dialogs 7 (5), 669–681.

Bird, J., 1993. Coming out of the closet: illuminating the therapeutic relationship. Journal of Feminist Theory 3 (5), 47–64.

Campbell, A.V., 1984. Moderated love: A theology of professional care. SPCK, London.

Cawthorn, A., 2006. Working with the denied body. In: Mackereth, P., Carter, A. (Eds.), Massage and bodywork: adapting therapies for cancer care. Elsevier, Edinburgh.

Cawthorn, A., Fielding, J., 2006. The DIRECT/Negotiation model poster

presentation. In: International Cancer Nursing Conference, Toronto.

Cunningham, A.J., 2000. The healing journey: overcoming the crisis of cancer. Key Porter Books, Toronto.

Ebell, H., 2008. The therapist as a travelling companion to the chronically ill: hypnosis and cancer related symptoms. Contemporary Hypnosis 25 (1), 46–56.

Erickson, M.H., Rossi, E.L., Rossi, S.I., 1976. Hypnotic realities: the induction of clinical hypnosis and forms of indirect suggestion. Irvington, New York.

Erskine, R.G., Moursund, J.P., Tratumann, R.L., 1999. Beyond empathy. A therapy of contact-in-relationship. Brunner/Mazel, Philadelphia.

Gehrie, M., 1999. On boundaries and intimacy in psychoanalysis. Progress in Self Psychology 15, 83–84.

Griffin, J., Tyrell, I., 2003. Human givens: a new approach to emotional health and clear thinking. Human Givens, Chalvington.

Hammond, D., 1984. Myths about Erickson and Ericksonian hypnosis. Am. J. Clin. Hypn. 26, 236–245.

Hayley, J., 1973. Uncommon therapy: the psychiatric techniques of Milton H Erickson MD. Norton, New York.

Hayley, J., 1985. Conversations with Milton H. Erickson MD, Vol. 1: Changing individuals. Norton, New York.

Heap, M., Aravind, K.K., 2002. Hartland's medical and dental hypnosis, fourth ed. Churchill Livingstone, Edinburgh.

Hobson, R., 1985. Forms of feeling: the heart of psychotherapy. Tavistock, London.

Horvarth, A.O., Bedi, R.P., 2002. The alliance. In: Norcross, J.C. (Ed.), Psychotherapy relationships that work. Oxford University Press, New York.

Horvarth, A.O., Symonds, B.D., 1991. Relation between working alliance and outcome in psychotherapy: a meta-analysis. Journal of Counselling Psychology 38, 139–149.

Howe, D., 1999. The main change agent in psychotherapy is the relationship between therapist and client. In: Feltman, C. (Ed.), Controversies in psychotherapy and counselling. Sage, London.

Johns, C., 2004. Being mindful easing suffering. Jessica Kingsley, London.

Jones, A., 1997. Death, poetry, psychotherapy and clinical supervision (the contribution of psychodynamic psychotherapy to palliative care nursing). J. Adv. Nurs. 25, 238–244.

Kirsch, I., 1990. Changing expectations: a key to effective psychotherapy. Brooks/Cole, Pacific Groves.

Kirsch, I., 1997. Response expectancy theory and application: a decennial review. Applied and Preventative Psychology 6, 69–79.

Lambert, M., Barley, D.E., 2001. Research summary on the therapeutic relationship and psychotherapy outcome. Psychotherapy: Theory, Research, Practice, Training 38 (4), 351–361.

Lambert, M.J., Okiishi, J.C., 1997. The effects of the individual psychotherapist and implications for future research. Clinical Psychology: Science and Practice 4, 66–75.

Lankton, S., Lankton, C., 1983. The answer within: a clinical framework of Ericksonian hypnotherapy. Brunner/Mazel, New York.

Lazarus, A.A., 1971. Behaviour therapy and beyond. McGraw-Hill, New York.

Lynn, S., Hallquist, M., 2004. Toward a scientifically based understanding of

Milton H. Erickson's strategies and tactics: hypnosis, response sets and common factors in psychotherapy. Contemporary Hypnosis 21 (2), 63–78.

Moursand, J.P., Erskine, R.G., 2003. Integrative psychotherapy: the art and science of relationship. Brooks/Cole, London.

Nuttall, J., 2002. Modes of therapeutic relationship in brief dynamic psychotherapy. A case study. Psychodynamic Practice 8 (4), 505–523.

O'Connor, J., 2001. NLP Workbook: a practical guide to achieving the results you want. Thorsons, Berwick-on-Tweed.

Orlinsky, D.E., Graves, K., Parks, B.K., 1994. Process and outcome in psychotherapy. In: Bergin, A.E., Garfield, S.L. (Eds.), Handbook of psychotherapy and behaviour change. Wiley, New York, pp. 257–310.

Overholser, J.C., 1988. Applied psychological hypnosis: management of problematic situations. Professional Psychology Research and Practice 19, 405–415.

Parle, M., Maguire, P., Heaven, C., 1997. The development of a training model to improve the health professionals skills, self-efficacy, outcome expectancies, when communicating with cancer patients. Soc. Sci. Med. 44 (2), 231–240.

Patterson, C.H., 1985. The therapeutic relationship: foundations for an eclectic psychotherapy. Brooks/Cole, Pacific Grove.

Rowan, J., 1998. Linking its place in therapy. International Journal of Psychotherapy 3, 245–254.

Safran, J.D., 1993. Breaches in the therapeutic alliance: an arena for negotiating authentic relatedness. Psychotherapy 30, 11–24.

Samuels, A., 1993. The political psyche. Sage, London.

Seigal, B.S., 2001. Peace, love and healing. Quill, New York.

Shaw, R., 2004. The embodied psychotherapist: an exploration of the therapist's somatic phenomena within the therapeutic encounter. Psychotherapy Research 14 (3), 271–288.

Short, D., Erickson, A.A., Klein, R.E., 2005. Hope and resiliency: understanding psychotherapeutic strategies of Milton H. Erikson. John Wiley, London.

Spanos, N.P., Coe, W.C., 1992. A social-psychological approach to hypnosis. In: Fromm, M.R., Nash, M.R. (Eds.),

Contemporary hypnosis research. Guildford Press, New York.

Tansy, M.J., Burke, W.F., 1989. Understanding countertransference: from projective identification to empathy. The Analytic Press, Hillsdale.

Yapko, M.D., 1992. Hypnosis and the treatment of depression: strategies for change. Brunner/Mazel, New York.

Yapko, M.D., 2001. Treating depression with hypnosis integrating cognitive, behavioural and strategic approaches. Brunner-Routledge, Florence.

Yapko, M.D., 2003. Trancework: an introduction to the practice of clinical hypnosis, third ed. Brunner-Routledge, New York.

FURTHER READING

Norcross, J.C. (Ed.), 2002. Psychotherapy relationships that work. Oxford University Press, New York.

Short, D., Erickson, B.A., Erickson Klein, R., 2005. Hope and resiliency: understanding the psychotherapeutic strategies of Milton H Erickson. Crown House, London.

USEFUL RESOURCES

www.hypno-therapist.com.
www.hypnosisaudio.com/scripts.htm.

www.hypnotherapyscripts.co.uk.
www.learnzone.macmillan.org.uk.

Working with the therapeutic relationship

6

Progressive muscle relaxation: a remarkable tool for therapists and patients

Peter A. Mackereth • Lynne Tomlinson

CHAPTER OUTLINE

Abbreviated progressive muscle relaxation training (APMRT), referred to more simply as PMR, is an established therapeutic technique used in stress and anxiety management by clinical psychologists and other health professionals. PMR has been discussed in other chapters of this book. Here we present an overview of PMR development, a review of the research work, and a protocol that can be the basis for creating your own PMR practice.

KEY WORDS

Progressive muscle relaxation
Training
Adaptations
Research

INTRODUCTION

Numerous benefits have been claimed for relaxation training for a variety of health problems associated with stress and anxiety, with a body of research work to its credit (Freeman 2001); this will be reviewed in more detail later in this chapter. Edmund Jacobson, the originator of the progressive muscle relaxation training, had observed in 1905 that deeply relaxed students demonstrated no obvious startle response to sudden noise; this became his life work (Jacobson 1977). He developed a lengthy and meticulous technique,

© 2010 Elsevier Ltd.
DOI: 10.1016/B978-0-7020-3082-6.00008-3

which focused on getting in touch with musculature and learning to control the tension levels. Jacobson's method was designed so that the practitioner would eventually be able to automatically and unconsciously monitor and release unwanted tension. The process has since been adapted and shortened by others, most notably Joseph Wolpe, and has become known as the abbreviated progressive muscle relaxation training. Included in this adaptation is the tension–release cycle (e.g. make a tight fist and then release) combined with a focus on breathing. This variation is part of Wolpe's framework called systematic desensitization, aimed at getting in touch with the individual's tension and the body's response, and then letting it go in a controlled manner. Freeman (2001) suggests that PMR and other muscle-based relaxation variations convey health benefits in three ways:

1. Utilizing the effects of PMR to manipulate autonomic responses
2. Increases or activates the production of opiates
3. Promotes optimal immune function.

Autonomic responses determine whether the body needs to engage in a 'fight-or-flight' or 'rest-and-digest' scenario or to a state somewhere between these two extremes. The sympathetic division of the autonomic nervous system (ANS), associated with 'flight-or-fight' responses, mobilizes the body in emergency and stressful circumstances. Many of these responses are not immediately apparent to our consciousness. Physically, blood flow is redirected away from the digestive process to the smooth muscle, heart rate and blood pressure increase, with these processes triggered by the increase of circulating catecholamines, which include adrenaline and noradrenaline (Hucklebridge & Clow 2002). Associated with the stress response is the release of cortisol, which mobilizes energy reserves, increases sensitivity of tissues to neurotransmitters and inhibits the immune and inflammatory response. Freeman (2001) argues that PMR techniques blunt sympathetic arousal by training the individual to reduce oxygen requirements, achieved by the repetitive release of muscle tension combined with slowing of respirations. This makes it a useful therapeutic intervention for panic, phobias and anxiety states.

Important to well-being, endogenous opioids, such as enkephalins, dynorphins, endomorphins and β-endorphin, have been found to have a variety of effects, including analgesic, anti-inflammatory and bronchodilation (Jessop 2002). These compounds and their receptor sites have been located within immune tissues (Stephanou et al 1990). It has been argued that opioids play an important part in modulating stress responses. It has been noted that opioid production is increased in adults who exercise regularly (Freeman 2001) and is reduced in adults with enduring health problems such as chronic fatigue syndrome (Conti et al 1998). In a laboratory experiment ($n = 32$) to determine the role of endogenous opioids in the effects of PMR training, McCubben et al (1996) found that PMR significantly reduced diastolic pressure, but when an opioid blockade was administered, it antagonized the PMR training. Hypnotherapists could utilize the potential responses of reduced anxiety and pain relief in the development of anchors and post-hypnotic suggestions, with an intention to help build a patient's resources (Box 6.1).

Over three decades, Herbert Benson and colleagues (1984) have investigated the psychological and physiological effects associated with the

BOX 6.1 Practice points

- Keep the delivery of this profound technique simple and slow – do less ... well
- Consider extending your perception and use of PMR as a therapist. As well as suggested uses in this chapter, PMR can be a kinesthetic induction, rapid re-induction, deepener and offers many opportunities to anchor positive resource states and can act as a link to post-hypnotic suggestions
- Consider adapting the PMR script – short versions can be used prior to hypnotherapy or as homework
- Introduce the session giving key benefits to the patient – these can be linked to his/her individual needs and are in themselves potential hypnotic suggestions
- Humour and visual imagery can be used to draw in, engage with a resource state and build rapport – the session should not be overly technical as this can reinforce rather than alleviate anxiety
- Consider closing the session with general and specific post-hypnotic suggestions
- Consider using PMR to help a patient regain full consciousness at the close of a hypnotherapy session – this can help to bring focus and grounding back to the body.

KEY CONCEPTS

relaxation response, elicited from PMR, meditation, yoga and physical exercise routines, many of which appear to be the opposite of the stress response. Stefano et al (1996: 3) have acknowledged that repetition is crucial to the relaxation response, but surmise that 'trust or belief in expected outcomes' can help to regulate immunological function via cognitive and neurological processes. This sense of improved well-being associated with the relaxation response has been labelled 'remembered wellness', which Benson (1996) has ascribed to memories of nurturance and maternal attachment. Lazar et al (2000) have investigated the relaxation response to meditation with functional magnetic resonance imaging (MRI) and mapped areas of the brain, which are responsive to opioids. Stefano et al (1996) suggests that this work demonstrates the mind–body wiring that could modulate the relationship between cognitive and physiological processes. In this review of neural processes and the relaxation response, Stefano and colleagues (1996) note that increased circulatory levels of opioids improve mood and sense of well-being, and refer to earlier work on enkephalins, which they found to have the additional benefit of stimulating immune cells. Aside from effects of opioids on heart rate, blood pressure, respiration, immune cells and mood, these compounds have also been found to stimulate antibacterial peptides in human studies (Tasiemski et al 2000). This information can provide a wealth of ideas for hypnotherapists using PMR and tailored suggestions, to enable patients to connect with feelings of being nurtured and supported.

The PMR method has a strong record of clinical efficacy and is an acknowledged standard strategy for a number of somatic states, including anxiety and stress, and features as part of clinical training in psychology (Pawlow & Jones 2002, Turner et al 1992). It is recommended that patients receive individual live instruction; indeed Lehrer and Woolfolk (1994) have argued that one-to-one training is crucial to effective training as well as any evaluative research. Relaxation techniques are increasingly being used as a non-pharmacological intervention by nurses, occupational therapists and medical practitioners in a variety of healthcare settings. DeMarco-Sinatra (2000), a nurse practitioner in the USA, believes that teaching relaxation techniques can be an appropriate role for nurses in both in-patient and out-patient settings. He argues that the activity supports patient autonomy and is cost-effective as a method of health promotion. We argue here that PMR and other forms of relaxation training are valuable additions to the hypnotherapy toolbox. Aside from being part of standard hypnotherapy induction training, PMR skills need to be updated and developed in ongoing training and supervision.

RESEARCH WORK

Many studies have investigated relaxation techniques; these have included imagery, guided relaxation and more structured techniques, such as PMR. Variations of PMR have developed, including the Mitchell Method, which involves body postures that are opposite to the physical responses to stress and anxiety (e.g. fingers spread rather than clenched). In autogenic relaxation training, the focus is on experiencing physical sensations in different parts of the body (e.g. heaviness or warmth) as a learnt sequence. Creative imagery and visualization techniques are also commonly described as relaxation techniques, and although they can be guided by pre-recorded audiotape guidance or a facilitator, any visual suggestions (e.g. beach or paradise setting) are usually interpreted and developed by the patient (Vickers & Zollman 1999). In practice (and in many of the studies located), some of the relaxation techniques described are a combination of techniques (e.g. 25 min of PMR ending with 5 min of imagery) or are not fully described in the research reports, making it difficult to evaluate their individual clinical effectiveness or otherwise.

There is early literature documenting the beneficial effects of PMR training in experimental studies on both psychological states and physiological functioning. For example, studies have found reduced sympathetic nervous system activity and cortisol levels following PMR training (McGrady et al 1987). Since then, a further 13 clinical studies have been conducted examining the immunological effects of PMR training. Some results are contradictory. For example two studies found there were no effects on white blood cells following PMR sessions (Peavey et al 1985, Hall et al 1993) while in contrast McGrady et al (1992) reported a decrease in white blood cells (WBCs) and neutrophils. Carlson and Hoyle's (1993) review of the PMR literature has concluded that providing the instruction in a one-to-one situation was more effective than with a group. Devine and Westlake (1995) conducted a meta-analysis of 116 studies involving patients who have cancer, with statistically significant reductions reported for levels of anxiety, depression, mood, pain, nausea, vomiting and pain. In clinical practice, PMR and other relaxation techniques, have been used for a number of years as supportive interventions for patients living with cancer (Sloman 2002), managing chemotherapy-related nausea and vomiting (Molassiotis 2000) and coping with chronic pain (Seers 1993).

In assessing the benefits of relaxation for chronic pain, Carroll and Seers (1998) conducted a systematic review. They included only controlled trials with 10 or more participants per treatment arm. The studies were assessed for methodological quality using a modified 3-item scale (Jadad et al 1996). Four studies in the review showed significant differences favouring relaxation for within-session changes, compared with no treatment controls. PMR was used in six of the studies mostly using audio-taped instruction. In Sloman's (1995) oncology study ($n = 67$) a significant difference was found for the 'live' relaxation vs 'no treatment' group for a pain sensation visual analogue scale. In one of the larger chronic pain studies ($n = 75$) reviewed, Seers (1993) again using 'live' rather than audio-taped PMR instruction vs control, two groups reported a significant difference for pain and anxiety, favouring PMR. The reviewers concluded that there was not enough conclusive evidence for a direct effect of relaxation techniques on chronic pain, but suggest that effects on coping and anxiety may contribute to the overall well-being of patients living with chronic pain. A second systematic review by Carroll and Seers (1998) of relaxation techniques, examined outcomes for patients with acute pain. Only seven (362 patients) out of a possible 40 studies were eligible for inclusion using the modified Jadad et al (1996) scale. When considering pain outcomes, only three out of the seven reported significantly less pain in the relaxation groups.

RECENT STUDIES

In a clinical study, Cheung et al (2001) assessed the effects of PMR training on anxiety and quality-of-life with patients ($n = 18$) after stoma surgery. There were significant differences for the PMR group with lower anxiety (C-STAI) scores than the control group. There was also a significant difference in the physical health/independence and general perception of the World Health Organization Quality of Life Scale (WHOQoL) with the experimental group reporting better functioning. There were no significant differences between the groups for change in a Quality of Life Index for Colostomy (QoL–Colostomy). The PMR sessions ranged from 11–20 for 20 min per week and were continued at home using an audiotape. It was necessary to adapt PMR for the experimental group to minimize the risk of peristomal hernia by avoiding tensing the abdominal muscles. Importantly, the first two postoperative sessions were supervised, with the patients then instructed to practice PMR at home 2–3 times per week after discharge. Patients were also asked to maintain a record of their PMR practice.

In a randomized controlled experimental study of PMR by Pawlow and Jones (2002), participants ($n = 46$) were led through two live sessions of PMR training. A further 15 control participants experienced two sessions of quiet sitting. Heart rate, state anxiety (SAI), perceived stress and salivary cortisol levels were examined twice. Participants returned 1 week later for a second session under the same conditions. Statistically significant changes in the experimental group in all measures were consistent across both sessions.

Sloman (2002) tested the efficacy of PMR and guided imagery for the alleviation of anxiety and depression in patients ($n = 56$) with advanced cancer. There were four treatment conditions: (1) PMR, (2) guided imagery (GI),

(3) PMR and GI, and (4) control group-standard care. The inclusion criteria excluded patients who had used the techniques before and only included patients assessed as emotionally distressed by a clinician. Each patient was visited twice a week for 3 weeks by a nurse, who remained with them while they listened to a tape of the technique(s) being played. Participants were encouraged to use the tapes, if possible daily, but details of how this was monitored were not reported. There were no significant difference between the techniques with measures of anxiety and depression (HADS), and a quality-of-life measure. Compared with the control group, there were significant differences for all three treatments for depression and quality-of-life, but only a borderline significant effect with anxiety ($p = 0.057$).

In Hernandez-Reif et al's (2002) pilot study, the effects of 10 massage therapy sessions vs 10 PMR sessions on disease-related symptoms and biochemical levels in individuals ($n = 16$) with Parkinson's disease (PD) were evaluated. After receiving the interventions twice a week for 5 weeks, the self-ratings improvements were statistically significant on an Activities of Daily Living Scale. Both groups reported more effective sleep, but the massage group had statistically significant less sleep disturbance than the PMR group. By the end of the 5 weeks, the massage group had statistically significant lower noradrenaline and adrenaline levels. An interesting finding was a statistically significant increase in urinary dopamine and epinephrine levels for the PMR group. Carrying out the PMR was reported as being stressful, possibly accounting for the rise in adrenaline; this may have been related to fatigue and difficulties with coordination associated with PD. However, an increase in dopamine levels was judged as encouraging, given that progressive PD is usually associated with lowering of the dopamine levels (Tekumalla et al 2001).

Using a quasi-experimental study by Sheu et al (2003), patients with essential hypertension were block assigned to either PMR or to a 'usual care' control group. Over a 4-week period, the intervention group attended a PMR training session and were asked to practice at home daily. There were immediate significant effects on pulse (weeks 1–4), systolic pressure (weeks 1–3 only) and diastolic pressure (weeks 1, 2 and 4). The intervention group also showed improvements in perceived stress and health scales, which were significant compared with the control group.

More recently, Kwekkeboom et al (2008) compared patient's perceptions of the effectiveness of guided imagery and PMR interventions with changes in pain scores. These interviews were with a subset of participants ($n = 26$) of 40 participants who took part in a randomized controlled crossover trial. Group 1 received relaxation on day 1 and then imagery on day 2. Group 2 participated in imagery on day 1 and then relaxation on day 2. The length of both interventions (15 min) was considered by the participants as desirable. Both interventions were reported as helping to relieve pain for durations of between 30 and 45 min, with PMR being perceived as slightly more effective than guided imagery.

Mackereth et al (2009) using a crossover design, compared outcomes for patients ($n = 50$) with multiple sclerosis, who received either reflexology first or second to compare therapeutic outcomes with weekly PMR training. Both interventions were provided for 6 weeks with a break of 4 weeks between the two phases of treatment. Both interventions had positive effects on a range of outcome measures (salivary cortisol levels, state anxiety inventory, short form SF–36, and General Health Questionnaire 28, heart and blood pressure recordings). Changes in cortisol levels pre-1st and post-6th sessions favoured reflexology, however post-session systolic blood pressure favoured PMR.

SAFETY ISSUES

Reports of concerns about PMR training are extremely rare. A survey was conducted by Edinger and Jacobsen (1982) with 116 clinicians who had conducted PMR practice with an estimated 17 542 clients. Reported side-effects were: intrusive thoughts (15%), fear of losing control (9%), upsetting sensory experiences (4%), muscle cramps (4%), sexual arousal (2%) and psychotic symptoms (0.4%). An adverse reaction to PMR practice has been described as relaxation-induced anxiety (RIA) and is judged to be an extremely small risk. It is however recommended to monitor patients with a history of panic disorder or hyperventilation for signs of rising anxiety during PMR (Freeman 2001). It has been suggested that PMR can be modified for persons with neuromuscular disability that limit their control of voluntary muscles. This can be achieved, e.g. by noticing tense muscle areas, but not increasing the tensions further before releasing (Cautela & Groden 1978). Compliance has also been identified as a challenge in evaluating PMR outcomes, given that patients undertake the technique, once trained, at home and unsupervised (Hernandez-Reif et al 2001) (see Box 6.2).

PMR PRACTICE POINTS

PMR is a mobile 'no frills' intervention. It can either be facilitated in a single session by a therapist or through a series of 'training' sessions in a quiet therapy space. PMR can be used in noisy environments; indeed the

---

BOX 6.2 Training points

- Provide tailored information to the patient about how PMR can help
- Plan the training, assess learning style, and contract for follow-up sessions to evaluate progress and reinforce the skill
- Ensure that the patient knows she/he can choose to close their eyes and can ask for guidance at any point
- Monitor for eyes-open trance states and ensure patients emerge completely from trance
- Patients can choose to observe the trainer/therapist demonstrate the PMR protocol and join in when comfortable – this can help to alleviate performance anxiety and promote pacing, matching and rapport
- Therapists can record (observing safety issues, e.g. not using when driving) an audio-version of PMR
- In the training, reinforce that patients need to practice PMR regularly; this can be a short version, daily or longer sessions, once or twice per week.

physicality of the technique gives the patient something to direct his/her attention to in less than ideal conditions. Even though PMR can be useful in reducing the risk of vasovagal responses associated with panic and anxiety states, care needs to taken in making sure that the environment is safe and comfortable for the patient. The therapist needs to ensure that he/she is lying down or sitting with feet and legs elevated. Pillows may be needed to provide support, particularly for posture, limbs and joints and a blanket needs to be available for warmth and security. It is also helpful to have water at hand for both patient and therapist. It is advisable to turn off mobile telephones/pagers and request 'no interruptions' during the training session. A useful addition is the availability of 'squeezy balls' – these can help to anchor the training (they can be taken away to practice). They also offer a focus for the activity, and, if appropriate, gentle humour (see Ch. 7).

The literature review suggests that PMR and creative imagery make a good combination and are a powerful and helpful means of linking thought and body. This combination has been found to be particularly useful in stressful clinical situations, such as prior to, and during intravenous cannulation. It has also been found to be helpful in the making and securing of masks during radiotherapy to treat head and neck cancers (see Ch. 7). If used during a hypnotherapy session, suggestions can be given to practice not only at home, but also prior to stressful situations, as a means of recognizing and actively reducing tension. This promotes and reinforces the relaxation response, the hypnotherapy work, builds resilience and self-efficacy. For example suggestions can be woven into a PMR session, such as:

- Practicing PMR can help reduce tension and improve well-being
- Long after this session is over you can continue to experience and reinforce any of the positive things you have felt and learnt today
- During your sleep tonight – as you breathe out – your body will continue to relax more and more deeply – this will help you make the most of your sleep – and on waking, feel more refreshed and recuperated.

TRAINING POINTS

From the literature review there are some key issues to consider when planning, delivering and evaluating PMR over a series of sessions. A minimum of two sessions provides opportunities to reinforce; however, we suggest six sessions on a weekly basis, which is supported by our review of the research. It has also been suggested that patients can be guided to practice PMR on a daily basis. It may be that PMR, when practiced more frequently, can be carried out with fewer areas of body worked and for shorter periods. A basic protocol is provided in Figure 6.1. The purpose of progressive muscle training approach is to achieve a state of relaxation by contracting and relaxing muscles in sequence; each set of muscles being worked four times. The therapist instructs and guides the patient with what to do at each stage of the protocol.

PMR Protocol

We are going to move through the muscles of the body, tightening and relaxing various muscle groups. Before we begin, minimize all interruptions and make yourself as comfortable as you can. Lie down or recline in a comfortable chair. Uncross your legs, loosen tight clothing, and remove your shoes. Your arms can be placed comfortably at your sides. As you tighten one part of your body leave the other parts limp and relaxed. You should not tighten a muscle so hard that you experience discomfort or cramping. The goal of this technique is to recognize the difference between tension and relaxation.

First, I will explain which muscle group we will begin with and how to tighten it. When I say, 'begin', I invite you to tighten the muscle group while taking a deep breath in. Hold this position for 6–10 seconds, when I'll say, 'release', relax the muscle group and continue to breathe out for 6–10 seconds until I say 'OK'.

I invite you now to close your eyes, knowing you can open them at any point and observe me doing each part of the technique. I will now guide you through the relaxation process.

Feet
First, we're going to start with your feet by curling the toes, making all of the muscles in your feet really tight. Begin now while taking a deep breath in. Now breathe out and release. Notice how relaxed your toes can become.

OK. Now you're going to tighten your feet muscles again. I invite you to squeeze the muscles of your feet really tight. Begin now and breathe in.

And now breathe out and release. Concentrating on how nice and warm your toes feel.

OK. You're going to tighten your feet muscles again, this time concentrating on how tense your feet feel. Begin now and take a deep breath in.

Now breathe out and release. Let all of the tension in your feet and toes run out of your body while releasing your out breath.

(Repeat with the feet one more time.)

Calf
Now we're going to move on to the calf muscles. I'm going to ask you to squeeze your calf muscles really tight. You can do this by pulling you heels inward towards your body. Begin tightening your calf muscles now while taking a deep breath in.

FIG 6.1 Example of a basic PMR protocol.

(continued)

And now breathe out and release. Just let your calves hang free, completely relaxed.

OK. Now we're going to repeat the calf muscles. Make sure you squeeze them really tight, so your calves are almost as hard as rocks. Begin now and breathe in.

Now breathe out and release. Ridding you calves of all of the tension as you breathe out.

OK. And again, you're going to contract your calf muscles. Go ahead and breathe in.

And now breathe out and release. Pushing out all of the tightness that was built up in your calves.

(Repeat calves one more time.)

Thigh
Next we're going to do the thigh muscles. I'm going to ask you to press and constrict your thigh muscles so that they feel hard and tight. Begin tightening your thigh muscles now while taking a big breath in.

And now breathe out and release. Letting the tension melt out of your thighs.

OK. Now you're going to tighten your thigh muscles again. Make sure you're squeezing them really tight! Begin now and breathe in.

And now breathe out and release. Concentrating on your thighs feeling wobbly like jelly.

OK. Now we're going to repeat the thigh muscles again. Pressing them hard and tight, think about how tense your thighs feel. Take a big breath in and begin.

And now breathe out and release. Moving the tension out of your thighs with the breath that is leaving your body.

(Repeat thighs one more time.)

Abdomen
And now we're going to focus on the abdomen. I want you to compress your abdomen muscles, crunching them together. Push your stomach out and squeeze as tightly as you can. Begin now while breathing in.

And breathe out and release. Letting the tension run out of your body.

FIG 6.1—cont'd

(continued)

Progressive muscle relaxation

OK. Now you're going to tighten those abdomen muscles again, concentrating on how rigid and tense they feel. Start now and breathe in.

Now breathe out and relax. Letting all of the tension leave your body.

OK. You're going to squeeze your abdomen muscles again, scrunching them up really tight. Breathe in and begin now.

And breathe out and release. Thinking about how relaxed your abdomen muscles feel now.

(Repeat one more time.)

Hands

Now we're going to move on to your hands. Tighten and curl your fingers into fists. Squeeze these fists so that you can feel the tension in them. Breathe in and begin now.

And breathe out and release. Letting the tension run out of your fingertips.

OK. And now you're going to tighten your hands again, clenching your fists so that they are really tight. Begin now while taking a deep breath in.

And now breathe out and release. Letting your hands lay limply in your lap.

OK. And again, you're going to squeeze all of the muscles in your hands. Contracting them so that they feel really tight. Breathe in and begin tightening your hands now.

And breathe out and release. Think about how loose and warm your hands feel.

(Repeat)

Arms

Now I'm going to ask you to make your arm muscles really tight. Contract your forearms and biceps so that they are hard, almost like rocks. Begin now and breathe in.

Now breathe out and release. Letting the tension out of your body.

OK. Now I want you to squeeze all of the muscles in your arms again. Concentrating on how tense your arms feel. Take a deep breath in and begin.

Now breathe out and release. Let your arms hang freely from your shoulders.

OK. And begin, you're going to tighten and contract those arm muscles. Squeezing them really tight. Begin now while breathing in.

FIG 6.1—cont'd

(continued)

And breathe out and release. Thinking about how nice and relaxed your arms feel.

(Repeat)

Back

And now we're going to concentrate on the muscles in your back. I'm going to ask you to tighten the muscles in your back. You can do this by pulling your shoulders back. Begin now while talking a deep breath in. Breathe out and release.

OK. Now you're going to tighten the muscles in your back again. Begin now and breathe in.

And breathe out and release. Letting the tension flow out of your body along with your breath.

OK. You're going to contract all of the muscles in your back again, squeezing them so that they are comfortably tight. Take a deep breath in and begin.

And breathe out and release. Relaxing the muscles in your back.

(Repeat)

Face

And now we're going to finish up with the face. I'm going to ask you to tighten all of the muscles in your face. Crease your brow and frown. Scrunch up all of the muscles in your face. Begin now while breathing in.

And now breathe out and release. Ridding your face of all of the tension while breathing out.

OK. Now you're going to tighten those face muscles again, squeezing them really tight. Begin.

And breathe out and release. Letting all of the strain and tightness run out of your face.

OK. And again, we're going to concentrate on those facial muscles. Begin tightening and breathe in. And breathe out and release. Completely relaxing your face while gently pushing your breath out.

(Repeat)

You have now completed your relaxation session. Remember what we have worked on – we started with the feet, then the calves, thighs, tummy, hands, arms, back and face.

FIG 6.1—cont'd

It is essential to assess for any contraindications to PMR training (e.g. unable to consent) or for adapting PMR training to accommodate healthcare problems (e.g. hearing impaired). The session should be paced, building in pauses and acknowledging achievement of the person's progress through the protocol. Hearing a calm voice and focusing the mind on carrying out the instructions can be enough to induce a relaxed and receptive state, quickly and easily. Training sessions provide opportunities for patients to become accustomed to being invited to relax, guided by a skilled therapist. A PMR training CD, recorded by the therapist, provides an opportunity to link and reinforce the supported sessions when a patient practices PMR independently. This supports, but does not replace, initial one-to-one training and can be individualized to include suggestions specific to the patient's needs. Mindful attention to the body can be a diversion from everyday thoughts and preoccupations – with the patient becoming more and more preoccupied with listening, internalizing and carrying out the instructions. It is always useful, early on in the training session to suggest:

Any mental chatter can be given permission to be present, gently acknowledged and then, when you are ready, return attention to the sound of my voice.

Again, any personalized CD recording or written guidance can include a similar statement.

CONCLUSION

The review of PMR research work was selective given the wealth of work to date; it suggests that PMR alone has beneficial effects and adding another technique, such as creative imagery, may accrue additional benefits. PMR can be a tool for both hypnotherapists and patients. As a therapeutic tool it can help focus attention and provide a resource in situations that trigger anxiety and panic. The practitioner needs to become competent in not only providing the training but also monitoring the practice with patients (Box 6.3). Importantly, there is a need to evaluate therapeutic outcomes for using PMR as an adjunct with hypnotherapy practice.

BOX 6.3 Practitioner development points

- Review your training in PMR and related teaching skills – to ensure that you are competent and confident to include it within your role and therapeutic repertoire
- Establish/contribute towards PMR policy and standard operating procedures where the service is provided within healthcare settings
- Consider evaluating your work formally – there is paucity of quality audit, service evaluation and research work on PMR as a hypnotherapy adjunct
- Receive ongoing supervision, and where appropriate, managerial support for the provision of this intervention with patients receiving medical care.

Benson, H., 1984. Beyond the relaxation response. Times Books, New York.

Benson, H., 1996. Timeless healing: the power of biology and belief. Scribner, New York.

Carlson, C.R., Hoyle, R.H., 1993. Efficacy of abbreviated progressive muscle relaxation training: a quantitative review of behavioural medicine research. J. Consult. Clin. Psychol. 61 (6), 1059–1067.

Carroll, D., Seers, K., 1998. Relaxation for the relief of chronic pain: a systematic review. J. Adv. Nurs. 27, 476–487.

Cautela, J.R., Groden, J., 1978. Relaxation: a comprehensive manual for adults, children, and children with special needs. Research Press, Champaign.

Cheung, Y.L., Molassiotis, A., Chang, A.M., 2001. A pilot study on the effect of progressive muscle relaxation training of patients after stoma surgery. Eur. J. Cancer Care (Engl) 10, 107–114.

Conti, F., Pittoni, V., Sacerdote, P., et al., 1998. Decreased immunoreactive β-endorphin in mononuclear leucocytes from patients with chronic fatigue syndrome. Clinical Experimental Rheumatology 16, 729–732.

DeMarco-Sinatra, J., 2000. Relaxation training as a holistic nursing intervention. Holist. Nurs. Pract. 14 (3), 30–39.

Devine, E.C., Westlake, S., 1995. The effects of psych-educational care provided to adults with cancer: meta-analysis of 116 studies. Oncol. Nurs. Forum 22, 1369–1381.

Edinger, J.D., Jacobsen, R., 1982. Incidence and significance of relaxation treatment side effects. Behav. Ther. 5, 137.

Freeman, L.W., 2001. Research on mind-body effects. In: Freeman, L.W., Lawlis, G.F. (Eds.), Complementary & alternative medicine: a research-based approach. Mosby, London.

Hall, H.R., Minnes Olness, K., 1993. The psychophysiology of voluntary immunomodulation. Int. J. Neurosci. 69, 221–234.

Hernandez-Reif, M., Field, T., Krasnegor, J., et al., 2001. Lower back pain is reduced and range of motion increased after massage therapy. Int. J. Neurosci. 105, 131–145.

Hernandez-Reif, M., Field, T., Largie, S., et al., 2002. Parkinson's disease symptoms are differentially affected by massage therapy vs. progressive muscle relaxation: a pilot study. Journal of Bodywork and Movement Therapy 6 (3), 177–182.

Hucklebridge, F., Clow, A., 2002. Neuroimmune relationship in perspective. In: Clow, A., Hucklebridge, F. (Eds.), Neurobiology of the immune system. Academic Press, London.

Jacobson, E., 1977. The origins and development of progressive relaxation. J. Behav. Ther. Exp. Psychiatry 8, 119.

Jadad, A.R., Moore, R.A., Carroll, D., et al., 1996. Assessing the quality of reports randomised controlled trials: is blinding necessary? Control. Clin. Trials 17, 1–12.

Jessop, D.S., 2002. Neuropeptides: modulators of immune responses in health and disease. In: Clow, A., Hucklebridge, F. (Eds.), Neurobiology of the immune system. Academic Press, London.

Kwekkeboom, K.L., Hau, H., Wanta, B., et al., 2008. Patients' perceptions of the effectiveness of guided imagery and progressive muscle relaxation interventions used for cancer pain. Complement. Ther. Clin. Pract. 14, 185–194.

Lazar, S.W., Bush, G., Gollub, R.L., et al., 2000. Functional brain mapping of the relaxation response and meditation. Neuroreport 11 (7), 1581–1585.

Lehrer, P.M., Woolfolf, R.L., 1994. Principles and practice of stress management, second ed. Guildford Press, New York.

Mackereth, P., Booth, K., Hillier, V., et al., 2009. Reflexology and relaxation training for people with MS: a controlled trial. Complement. Ther. Clin. Pract. 15, 14–21.

McCubben, J.A., Wilson, J.F., Bruehl, S., et al., 1996. Relaxation training and opioids inhibition of blood pressure response to stress. J. Consult. Clin. Psychol. 64 (3), 593–601.

McGrady, A., Woerner, M., Bernal, G.A.A., et al., 1987. Effects of biofeedback assisted relaxation on blood pressure and cortisol levels in normotensives and hypertensives. J. Behav. Med. 10, 301–310.

McGrady, A., Conran, P., Dickey, D., et al., 1992. The effects of biofeedback-assisted relaxation on cell-mediated immunity, cortisol, and white blood cell count in healthy adult subjects. J. Behav. Med. 15, 343–354.

Molassiotis, A., 2000. A pilot study of the use of progressive muscle PMR training in the management of post-chemotherapy nausea and vomiting. Eur. J. Cancer Care (Engl) 9, 230–234.

Pawlow, L.A., Jones, G.E., 2002. The impact of abbreviated progressive muscle relaxation on salivary cortisol. Biol. Psychol 60, 1–16.

Peavey, B., Lawlis, F., Goven, A., 1985. Biofeedback assisted relaxation: Effects on phagocytic capacity. Biofeedback Self Regul. 10 (1), 33–47.

Seers, K., Maintaining people with chronic pain in the community: teaching relaxation as a coping skill. 1993. Department of Health, London. Department of Health Post-Doctoral Nursing Research Fellowship Report.

Sheu, S., Irvin, B.L., Lin, H.S., et al., 2003. Effects of progressive muscle relaxation on blood pressure and psychosocial status for clients with essential hypertension in Taiwan. Holist. Nurs. Pract. 17 (1), 41–47.

Sloman, R., 1995. Relaxation and the relief of cancer pain. Nurs. Clin. N. Am. 4, 697–709.

Sloman, R., 2002. Relaxation and imagery for anxiety and depression control in community patients with advanced cancer. Cancer Nurs. 25 (6), 432–435.

Stefano, G.B., Scharrer, B., Smith, E.M., et al., 1996. Opioid and opiate immunoregulatory processes. Critical Review in Immunology 16, 109–144.

Stephanou, A., Jessop, D.S., Knight, R.A., et al., 1990. Corticotropin-releasing factor-like immunoreactivity and mRNA in human leucocytes. Brain, Behaviour & Immunity 4, 67–73.

Tasiemski, A., Salzet, M., Benson, H., et al., 2000. The presence of opioids and antibacterial peptides in human plasma during coronary artery bypass surgery. J. Neuroimmunol. 109, 228–235.

Tekumalla, P.K., Calon, F., Rahman, Z., et al., 2001. Elevated levels of DeltaFosB and RGS9 in striatum in Parkinson's disease. Biol. Psychiatry 50, 55–74.

Turner, S.M., Calhoun, K.S., Adams, H.E. (Eds.), 1992. Handbook of clinical behavioral therapy. John Wiley, New York.

Vickers, A., Zollman, C., 1999. ABC of complementary therapies – hypnotherapy and relaxation therapies. Br. Med. J. 319, 1346–1349.

SECTION 2
APPROACHES IN CLINICAL PRACTICE

INTRODUCTION

Section 1 explored key concepts related to the underpinning evidence, models of practice and professional issues related to integrative practice. Section 2 focuses on the professional practice issues relevant to discreet areas of integrated and often innovative hypnotherapy work. As with the first section, some chapters are a team effort drawing on collaborative and complementary approaches to patient care. In each of the eight chapters in this section, the authors overview the approaches taken, examining key issues and concerns, supported by the available literature, anonymous case studies and reflective practice exercises. The practice areas discussed, although not exhaustive, are exemplars of evolving and valued work by therapists.

In Chapter 7, Peter A. Mackereth and Paula Maycock share their work with anxious patients who not only have a life-threatening medical diagnosis but who are coping with the challenges of investigations and treatments. They review hypnotherapy interventions from their own clinical practice, including nausea, needle phobia and panic through the use of case studies and illustrations.

In Chapter 8, Ann Carter and Peter A. Mackereth explore a range of therapeutic interventions which utilize 'hypnotic trance' to improve well-being and promote resilience in the face of illness or coping with loss. They discuss issues relating to safety and the importance of language and aftercare.

In Chapter 9, Anne Cawthorn and Kathy Stephenson explore these issues during health, illness, accident and following sexual abuse. A variety of assessment models and different hypnotherapeutic approaches are illustrated through the use of case studies.

In Chapter 10, Lynne Tomlinson, Paula Maycock and Peter A. Mackereth offer a very different approach to smoking cessation where the client and therapist work in harmony. A SEEDING model is presented and working this way is illustrated by case studies and reflective exercises.

In Chapter 11, Elisabeth Taylor discusses the development and provision of a combined hypnotherapy and cognitive therapy package offered to this patient group. Findings from this project are discussed, including participants' experiences and recommendations for training and development.

In Chapter 12, Kathy Stephenson explores a flexible practice model based on her extensive experience using hypnotherapy techniques with children. She covers a number of common problems such as enuresis, pain anxiety and low self-esteem.

In Chapter 13, Elisabeth Taylor explores the impaired quality of life and emotional distress which patients with these disorders experience. She discusses the published evidence supporting the clinical efficacy of various combinations of psychological therapies.

In Chapter 14, Anne Cawthorn, Bernadette Shepherd, Kevin Dunn and Peter A. Mackereth discuss this rewarding, yet challenging area for a therapist; which is working with patients who are coming to terms with their own mortality. They introduce the SERVICE model and suggest ways of working while being a companion to the person who is undertaking his/her own existential journey.

Anxiety and panic states: the CALM model

Peter A. Mackereth • Paula Maycock

7

CHAPTER OUTLINE

When faced with a life-threatening medical diagnosis, challenging investigations and treatments, patients and sometimes their carers, can respond by exhibiting distress, anxiety and panic states. This chapter explores the concept of anxiety and reviews hypnotherapy interventions that can be of value in acute care situations. Case studies are used to explore medical procedural anxiety, including nausea, needle phobia and panic. Additionally, practice points for healthcare professionals are included.

KEY WORDS

Distress
Anxiety
Panic
Phobias
CALM model
Interventions

ation

© 2010 Elsevier Ltd.
DOI: 10.1016/B978-0-7020-3082-6.00009-5

INTRODUCTION

It is impossible to live even an ordinary life without experiencing some form of stress. Major life events such as loss of a loved one, have been claimed to significantly affect health and well-being (Freeman 2001). Holmes and Rahe (1967) have categorized life events on the basis of the amount of life adjustment needed. Other authors have advocated that more commonplace stresses such as examinations, family arguments, transport difficulties and unexpected bills have a much larger summative impact on psychological states, outlook and well-being (Lazarus & Folkman 1989). Coe (1999) has identified different models, which attempt to explain the relationship between stress, immunity and disease:

1. Deterioration in health can occur as a result of cumulative or incremental stresses (critical thresholds)
2. Set points for changes in immunity may be triggered or lowered (critical periods)
3. Stressors may act as catalysts facilitating the action of a chain of immunological events (co-factors).

Fear, anxiety and other strong emotional states usually activate the sympathetic nervous division of the autonomic nervous system (ANS). Patients may present with acute stress, e.g. during a medical investigation, in addition to chronic states of stress linked to a long-term medical or mental health condition. Chronic states of anxiety and stress frequently cause increased muscle tension (tonus), reduction in peripheral skin temperatures and a hyperactive response to any further occurrence of an acute stressor. The individual can have difficulty being able to return to or maintain a hypoactive or relaxed state. The physical manifestations of the chronic state of arousal and constant state of low threshold to stressors can be seen in measurements of sympathetic nervous system (SNS) responses and physical complaints. For example the individual may be hypertensive, have reduced peripheral temperatures and report back and neck stiffness.

It is important for the therapist to have an understanding of the processes that are there to protect an individual physically (e.g. to run away from an imminent threat). In terms of responding physically to stress, the most direct brain pathway is the sympathetic-adrenal-medullary (SAM) axis. This pathway functions by activating the ANS. It does this by using informational substances, neurotransmitters and neuropeptides, which communicate directly with the immune system triggering changes at tissue and cellular level. The second and less direct brain pathway is the hypothalamic-pituitary-adrenal (HPA) axis. This pathway triggers the endocrine system to release hormones as informational substances. These in turn modulate both physiology and immunity. Henry (1986) attempted to define three types of physiological reactions linked to an emotional experience to articulate how they influence behaviour (Fig. 7.1).

The connections between the emotional state, disease processes and experience have been, and continue to be, explored in the emerging science of psychoneuroimmunology (PNI). This is the seminal work of Ader and Cohen (1975) and Ader (1982). This theory centres on a 2-way relationship

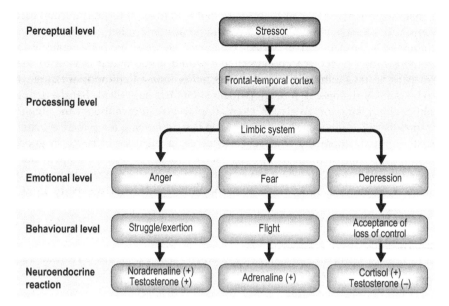

Perceptual level		Stressor	

FIG 7.1 Model of physiological reactions to stressors (Henry 1986).

between the immune system and the central nervous system (Rabin et al 1989, Lloyd 1990). Chemical as well as hormonal changes play a key part in the process of responding to stress. Aside from adrenaline and noradrenaline, cortisol is also produced. This steroid is necessary for raising glucose levels, and has anti-allergic and anti-inflammatory properties, needed in fight-or-flight situations. However, chronically elevated cortisol is associated with an increased risk of depression, diabetes and cancer (Sterling & Eyer 1992). It is inevitable that many patients living with these conditions will have frequent and sometimes lengthy contact with health professionals and services. Importantly for this chapter, these patients will be subject to numerous medical investigations, procedures and treatments.

Even in healthy individuals, researchers have identified immunological effects of stress. Medical students have reported more illness associated with examinations than at any other time during their training (Glaser et al 1987). Participants were found to show reductions in natural killer cells, thought to be integral in defence against viral infections and neoplastic growth, during examination periods (Kiecolt-Glaser 1984).

As therapists, our work is important not only for helping with acute stressors, but also assisting patients, and sometimes their carers, to manage chronic stress. There have been numerous studies that have examined psychoneuroimmunological outcomes of therapeutic interventions such as behavioural therapy, guided imagery, massage and progressive muscle relaxation (Groer & Ohnesorge 1993, Groer et al 1994, McCain et al 1994) (see Ch. 6). It can be concluded that interventions to affect emotional states can influence physiological states, which in turn can have immunological effects.

In this chapter we will overview various stress-related concepts and explore hypnotherapy and other strategies in acute situations, not only to assist the patients to master their stress, but also to learn techniques that can help in the longer term. Critics of hypnotherapy and other complementary therapies have labelled reported positive outcomes as being merely a demonstration of the placebo effect. We would argue that it is vital to see 'placebo' as a valuable therapeutic effect rather than an unimportant artefact to be quickly dismissed. Indeed, Benson (1996) has suggested that the act of physically taking or receiving even a 'placebo' intervention can trigger 'remembered wellness'. This process involves harnessing the patient's belief system, giving them the confidence to access a memory of being in good health or a time without symptoms. Benson believes that techniques that promote relaxation can be a good opportunity to access this innate resource since it provides a time to quieten the mind and assist the body in its own healing.

DEFINITIONS OF TERMS

ANXIETY

It is important to remember anxiety is a tool given by nature to make you cautious. The capacity to induce anxiety is a skill we all have for life. Importantly, anxiety is a subjective experience, which has significant physiological changes/responses, as well as behavioural features that affect how a person looks and acts. If anxiety persists, it can lead to depression.

PANIC

Panic is an extreme form of anxiety with marked ANS arousal (Box 7.1) leading to a need to remove oneself from the situation, i.e. 'run away'. Ignoring emerging feelings of panic does not help overcome it. The reactions are there to trigger the person to avoid harm. It is advisable to teach the patient to recognize his/her own panic responses and implement an intervention(s) suitable for him/her. It is important to acknowledge that the body cannot maintain a permanent state of panic.

BOX 7.1 Panic disorders signs and symptoms

- Spontaneous attack of intense fear
- Palpitations/sweating/tremors
- Shortness of breath
- Choking sensation
- Chest pain or discomfort
- Dizzy/lightheaded
- Fear of going crazy/dying
- Numbness, hot flashes, etc.
- Flashbacks of prior trauma
- Reversion to mother tongue
- Difficulty in comprehending complex instructions.

PHOBIA

This term is often used too glibly, with <4% of the population at risk from phobic reactions. Phobias have been classically defined by Choy et al (2007: 267) as 'characterized by an excessive, irrational fear of a specific object or situation, which is avoided at all cost or endured with great distress'. In terms of medical procedures, such as cannulation, it would be expected that the patient would quickly progress from a panic state to hyperventilating that would ultimately lead to a vasovagal reaction (Deacon & Abramowitz 2006).

WORKING WITH ANXIETY, PANIC AND PHOBIA STATES

It is very important to acknowledge that medical procedures can be extremely frightening for patients and their carers. Being cannulated repeatedly for blood sampling and/or for the administration of chemotherapy, particularly if unsuccessful can begin to become a feared event. Having your face covered in plaster or being clamped into position for radiotherapy (Fig. 7.2), even for short periods of time, can feel like being trapped. At the heart of the issue is feeling helpless and for some patients being reminded of previous episodes in their life when under threat or even being physically abused or raped.

A key to working with anxiety states is the construct of *locus of control*, first described by Rotter (1975). This has been measured using three subscales: external and internal loci of control and fatalism. Scores that are high on external locus are interpreted as the individual believing they have no or little control over their situation. Individuals scoring high on the internal locus of control subscale are described as having a sense of control and self-determination. It is important for therapists to recognize that individuals differ on how they personally control life situations, although certain psychosocial reactions, such as depression and anxiety are commonly reported among people living with life-threatening illness (Arias Bal et al 1991, Livneh & Antonak 1997). Interventions that can help to mitigate or alleviate acute stress can therefore be pivotal in assisting patients to maximize well-being, despite living with chronic and enduring illness. The interventions can also break the chains that lead some patients to develop anticipatory anxiety, panic states and phobic reactions. There are a number of possible co-factors that have been identified as contributing to this chain of events (Box 7.2). It is important for therapists/health professionals to be aware of these and assess patients exhibiting anxiety for risk.

Lazarus and Folkman's (1984) theoretical formulation differentiates between problem-focussed coping (i.e. strategies to alter stressful situations) and emotion-focussed coping (i.e. strategies to regulate feelings). For therapists and health professionals, there is a need to address both the problem and the reaction. For example, the problem might be venous access. Fear and anxiety will exacerbate this situation, with patients expressing the desire to escape and even withdraw from treatment as an 'in the moment' reaction. Sedating a patient may address the problem of the procedure, but not the feeling. In a study by Buelow (1991) investigating coping strategies,

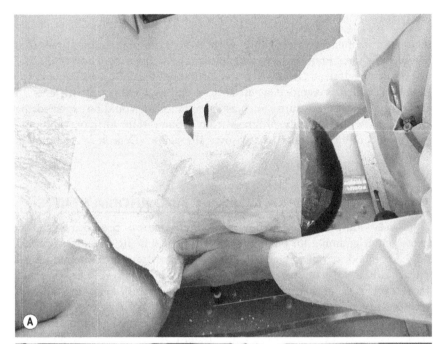

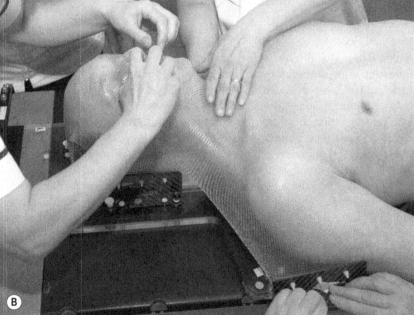

FIG 7.2 **Plaster cast** (A) for creating a mask and (B) a finished mask being fixed into position.

participant's depressions and feelings of uncertainty about the future, lead them to express preference for emotion-focussed strategies. Ignoring the emotional needs by using sedation alone, we are not meeting the whole person in their distress. The cycle repeats itself with every stressful procedure, so reinforcing the inability of the patient to have any measure of control.

BOX 7.2 Factors that may influence anxiety states

- Lower body weight
- First-time donors
- 'Fear of fainting'
- Concerns about health hazards
- Disgust
- Fear of fear
- Pain
- Medications – hypnotics, anxiolytics
- Smoking, alcohol and other substance misuse
- Younger age group: 13–19 adolescents.

Choy et al (2007), Wolitzky et al (2008).

BOX 7.3 Anxiety, panic and phobia states: concerns and risks

- Risk of injury from vasovagal reactions
- Non-compliance to treatment
- Increase staff time
- Sedation hazards, e.g. need to admit recovering patient, unable to drive, etc.
- Further conditioning of the phobia
- Stressful for carers
- Healthcare staff can feel guilt because the procedure/treatment/intervention appears to have triggered the panic
- Time constraints: next patient waiting to use the simulator/radiotherapy suite/mould room.

There are a number of risks and concerns when working with patients experiencing anxiety, panic and phobia states (Box 7.3). Aside from risks to the patient there are also repercussions for carers who can feel overwhelmed by seeing loved ones in so much distress. For staff repeatedly seeing acutely ill patients and their carers anxious and frightened contributes to 'burnout' (Iskihan et al 2004). Lacovides et al (2000) suggest that practitioners working in stressful clinical areas can acquire higher anxiety levels, performance disorders, and even symptomatology. Ethically, as well as economically, sedation presents problems, with a sedated patient less able to consent and needing greater recovery time, often requiring admission to hospital.

THE IMPORTANCE OF LANGUAGE

How information is relayed and the words chosen by health professionals are very influential in healthcare situations with patients and their carers. Failures to communicate effectively are a major cause of complaints from patients and their families. We live in an increasingly litigious world where patients, quite rightly, expect to be fully informed and consented prior to medical procedures, investigations and treatments. This presents a dilemma for professionals imparting information and answering a patient's or carer's questions. Health professionals, by word and by behaviour, can inadvertently promote further emotional and physical instability in patients. Much attention has been paid to the concept of placebo (Beecher 1955), yet the reverse is possible. The term 'nocebo' has been coined to refer to expectations of side-effects of treatment actually triggering symptoms to manifest and even be exhibited before a drug has fully entered the patient's system. Balancing the ethical duty to fully inform without feeding fears and promoting phobias is a major, but not insurmountable challenge.

ANXIETY-CONTROL STRATEGIES

There is some debate as to what are the best non-pharmacological approaches to reducing and/or managing anxiety. Clearly for patients wanting essential medical treatment avoiding the feared procedure is not a viable option. There are several options identified in the wider literature (Parrish et al 2008, Wolitzky-Taylor 2008), each requiring negotiation with the patient and involvement with the health professional, these include:

- Safety behaviour: The patient identifies something that has helped them in the past, e.g. I can only get through it with X, such as 'I need my mum with me' or 'I need medication the night before'. If the chosen safety behaviour fails, the patient may experience worsening anxiety
- Option to stop/move away/take a break. Offering this option instils an element of control for the patient. For the health professional this means that they need to able to stop a technical procedure and accommodate 'time out'
- Partial distractor: This may require an additional person who can engage the patient in conversation and talk them through the procedure. Rapport and effective communication skills are essential
- Moderate distractor: This activity should take significant attention and focus, however if anxiety is already surfacing, concentrating on a puzzle or word game may be too challenging
- Mastery activity: active engagement with body and thought processes during exposure. Here a technique such as progressive muscle relaxation or breathing technique could be used (see Ch. 6).

THE CALM MODEL

The CALM model (Box 7.4) proposed here is based on a service that evolved from a 2-year hypnotherapy project evaluated within an acute cancer care setting (see Ch. 11). The authors, together with the wider supportive care team, began offering one-to-one therapy sessions to patients prior to procedures/admission, as well as *in situ* intervention and support. The CALM model can encompass the aforementioned anxiety – control strategies, but what is unique is the availability of a therapist skilled in touch techniques and hypnotherapy. It could be argued that a healthcare professional (HCP) could provide part of this service. Indeed, mindful language and a calm presence can prevent worsening anxiety in patients. We argue that a therapist's

BOX 7.4 The CALM model for acute care situations

- Help patients to be Calm *now* – hold, nurture and ground
- Recognize anxiety – *teach* patients the signs and symptoms
- Regain and learn *control* – train *in situ*/rehearse in therapy sessions
- Use mindful and positive *language* – role model with therapists/healthcare professionals.

presence and skill can allow the HCP to concentrate on the procedure and the overall safety of the patient. The role of therapist is to be a skilled facilitator using a variety of therapeutic tools to best match the needs of the patient, both *in situ* and in preparing him/her for future procedures. Additionally, a therapist can assist a patient to process and/or clarify past triggers that have influenced current reactions to situations/procedures (see Case study 2, Box 7.6). It is important that therapists and health professionals, if concerned about a patient's mental health and possibility of self harm or suicidal intent or thought, make an urgent referral to a psychiatrist or psycho-oncology team.

HELP PATIENTS TO CALM *NOW*

Ideally, patients known to have procedure-related anxieties will have been offered hypnotherapy and/or stress management techniques prior to the event. However, in practice it is common for anxiety and panic states to begin immediately prior to a procedure. Patients may have attempted to conceal their anxiety and hoped that their feelings would diminish. If called to assist a patient during a procedure, the therapist, we suggest, should introduce him/herself with confidence, acknowledge the acute stress situation and then offer strategies to *regain control*. First, this can include guiding patients to moisten their mouth by moving the tongue around the gums or sipping lukewarm water. This simple technique for oral focus can comfort patients and contrasts with the discomfort of the 'anxious dry mouth'. Second, rather than draw attention to breathing (the patient may be hyperventilating), a therapist can guide the person to participate in active relaxation. Here it is very useful to offer a squeezy ball (Fig. 7.3) or similar compressible object. The therapist can demonstrate how to squeeze the ball and then observe the object regain its shape as the person breathes out gently and slowly.

An abbreviated form of progressive muscle relaxation (PMR) can be offered as a frontline technique to redirect the attention from wanting to take flight to actively tightening and releasing various muscle groups, repeating each area of the body four times. The therapists can engage physically with the patient and the PMR movements, e.g. asking the patient to push with feet against a held foam wedge or pillow. The therapist can also gently hold the patient's knees, asking him or her to visualize 'crushing walnuts' between them. We suggest that a patient works three or four areas such as the feet, knees, hands and shoulders over approximately 5–7 min. Only when the patient has begun to notice a change in his/her emotional and physical state

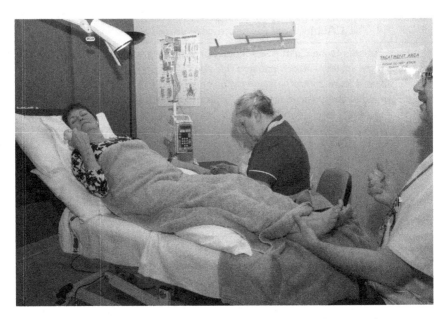

FIG 7.3 Squeezy ball being used combined with holding and guidance during cannulation.

can the procedure be consented for. Here again, patients can be reassured that they can take a break from the procedure at any point to repeat the PMR.

'AROMASTIX' AND HYPNOREFLEXOLOGY©

The following practice requires additional training in the use of aromatherapy and/or reflexology or a hypnotherapist and complementary therapist working together. First, taking aromatherapy, this can be offered in the form of 'aromastix' which contain a blend of plant essential oils held on a wick encased within a plastic tube. This tube is perforated to allow the aroma to escape as required when sniffed (Fig. 7.4). The prepared stick has an outer cover to limit the evaporation of the oils and make the stick portable and easy to use. When prepared by a trained aromatherapist, the essential oil blend can be customized to include oils with claimed benefit for alleviation of anxiety, nausea and insomnia (see Further Reading). The authors also use various blends to assist in smoking cessation work (see Ch. 10). It is possible to further modify the blends to include particular patient preferences for aroma, which maximizes compliance with this treatment. Provided in acute stress situations, aromastix can be used as a distractor, an anchor and a trigger to assist in rapid re-induction to a trance state.

The use of touch therapies, e.g. focusing on the feet, can be a safe and acceptable method of grounding a person in an acute state of anxiety or panic (see Ch. 8). HypnoReflexology© has been developed by the authors to bring together hypnotherapy with the art of reflexology (Maycock & Mackereth 2009). Case study 1 (Box 7.5) gives an example, with the therapist using reflexology to induce a trance state, and suggesting ways of reducing the intensity of nausea, thus enabling the patient to become calm and more focused.

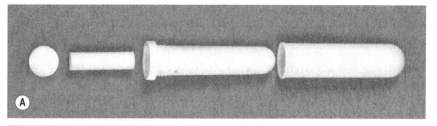

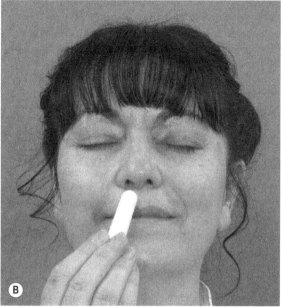

FIG 7.4 'Aromastix'. (A) The component parts with inner cotton wick and (B) in use.

BOX 7.5 Case study 1

Matthew aged 29 with renal cancer: 'My consultant says my tumour is responding well to the chemotherapy but I just can't stand the idea of any more needles. It's got worse with each treatment and now I panic for the week beforehand. The fear takes over my life. I can't function. I can't even go out and I don't sleep. I can't eat because I feel sick and this constant nausea is now overwhelming me. I can't stand it anymore'.

Matthew was refusing to continue with his chemotherapy at the time of the referral and was extremely distressed. A therapist offered to provide HypnoReflexology© as a means to enable him to calm down and travel home safely. He agreed and after 30 min his nausea dissipated and he reported feeling really 'chilled out'. This relief was a turning point for him. He decided that, with this help, he could stay and receive his chemotherapy that day. At the end of this treatment, the nurse asked Matthew how he would like to proceed. He asked for the therapist to be present during cannulation for his future treatments.

When Matthew finally left the chemo-suite, the nurse commented to the therapist 'I felt so relaxed listening to you and watching the foot massage that it relaxed me too . . . it made my job so much easier'.

Matthew completed his remaining treatments without distress.

BOX 7.6 Case study 2

Susan, aged 41, was scheduled for reconstructive surgery after treatment for breast cancer. In attending for preoperative assessment, Susan revealed a fear of hospitals, recounting having an anaesthetic mask being put on her face 10 years earlier and panicking, fearing she was going to die.

It was arranged for a therapist to meet Susan the day before surgery. She was tearful on arrival and was offered a gentle foot massage and hypnotherapy. Initially, the therapist explained that the response Susan had experienced was a normal response of her body to a fearful situation, which she found very reassuring. After 10 minutes, Susan was calmer. During trance state Susan chose an image of her mother sitting quietly holding and protecting her at all times during the hospital stay. The therapist suggested Susan talk freely with her anaesthetist about her concerns. The therapist and Susan planned with the anaesthetist that Susan could hold the mask and place it over her own face.

HELPING PATIENTS TO RECOGNIZE AND NORMALIZE ANXIETY

Ideally, treatment needs to be planned with the therapist meeting with the patient prior to the procedure. In a quiet therapy space, a patient can comfortably explore his/her concerns without the pressure of an imminent procedure. If called to support *in situ* helping patients to recognize and normalize anxiety begins straight away. Acknowledging that the various signs and symptoms the patient is experiencing is the body's normal way of going into survival mode (Case study 2, Box 7.6). An important part of the therapist's role is to explain the physical manifestations of stress and anxiety. The therapist can also reflect back the subtle changes in the patient's physical state when the relaxation process begins to occur. For example noticing change in the dilation of veins in the hand as the extremities warm up. Indeed, making suggestions that the arms, hands, legs and feet are feeling heavy and warmer can be helpful. During the out breath, patients can be invited to: '... let the shoulders drop down and then drop a little bit more', or when practising at home, suggest: 'scan your body for areas of tension and then with your out breath imagine that tension melting and softening, melting and softening'.

HELP PATIENTS TO REGAIN LOST CONTROL

Therapists can confidently suggest that panic will pass, indeed it is impossible to sustain, and to invite patients to notice when it settles. Any interventions need to be chunked down into smaller sections/stages. It is also essential to acknowledge success in every small way.

Guiding and training the patient in PMR can help the patient to shift the focus from being fearful and anxious to a calmer state (see Ch. 6). Case study 3 (Box 7.7) demonstrates the importance of following up the CALM *in situ* intervention with training sessions as the patient continued to receive daily radiotherapy. The therapist can create an audio-recording (tape, CD or MP3 recording) for the patient to continue the practice independently.

BOX 7.7 Case study 3

John, aged 35, was receiving daily radiotherapy for oral cancer. It was his 10th session and he was not tolerating wearing the mask. He said 'I would rather die than experience the fear of being locked into the treatment mask again' (Fig. 7.2). These feelings had been getting progressively worse from day one. Simply thinking about the sound of the mask being clicked into place was enough to make John struggle with his breathing, feel sick and light-headed and led him into panic.

Initially he was directed to moisten the mouth. He was then taught a simple PMR technique of tightening muscles in the hands and lower limbs. John worked each area four times in rotation, releasing tension with his out breath. During radiotherapy, this was reinforced by the therapist over the intercom system. He completed the treatment without becoming fearful. John was so impressed with this result that he arranged to see the therapist outside the session to learn self-hypnosis in combination with PMR, using a 'squeezy ball' to facilitate muscle contraction. The radiotherapist suggested that John bring his own music to play while using the PMR technique. John managed to complete all 25 remaining radiotherapy sessions.

MINDFUL LANGUAGE AND THERAPEUTIC PRESENCE

Information and language needs to be mindful and sensitive to the individual; purposively promoting understanding and emotional and physical stability. Humour can be used, but it must be appropriate. It is important to acknowledge the patient's success at every stage and reinforce and gently remind the patient to utilize learnt strategies. In anxiety states, patients can regress to the time of the original trigger or may have difficulty in comprehending complex terms and instructions. It is possible that patients move emotionally in panic states between child and adult states (see Ch. 12). Interventions that use nurturing can be helpful but health professionals and therapists alike must be careful not to automatically 'parent' the patient.

Healthcare professionals take the lead in procedures and need to be involved in reviewing with the patient, therapist and sometimes carers, as to what is helping and what other strategies can be offered. In Case study 3 (Box 7.7), the radiotherapist suggests 'John' chooses his own music and supports his practice of moistening of the mouth and PMR during the radiotherapy. It is very important that the patient sees and experiences their care being a team effort.

Intravenous cannulation can be a common trigger for anxiety (Box 7.8) and indeed can become linked with panic and in a small number of cases, patients become phobic (Cox & Fallowfield 2006). Patients can lose confidence in health professionals if the procedure is unsuccessful and/or painful. In practice, if two attempts are unsuccessful, the third can be done by another member of the team. Patients quickly attach to the HCP who successfully cannulates them the first time and will request the same person each time. Suggestions are made for those involved in this procedure in Box 7.9 to prevent cannulation-related anxieties.

BOX 7.8 Case study 4

Deborah, aged 36, with cervical cancer was receiving chemotherapy. She found cannulation increasingly difficult and for her third treatment session, a therapist was called to assist her. Deborah did not want a massage treatment as she was uncomfortable being touched. She was offered an 'aromastix' containing a blend of plant essential oils and was guided to inhale the aroma during a breathing/ relaxation exercise. This combination quickly created a 'pattern interrupt' in the session and assisted Deborah to enter a light trance state.

It was suggested to Deborah that: *'being so relaxed helps to dilate veins and so makes cannulation so much easier. Deborah you are in charge and can speak with the nurse or therapist at anytime you want'*. Then, 15 minutes into the creative imagery, Deborah quietly said, 'I am feeling really calm and can manage that needle now'. She laughed aloud when the nurse said 'it went in first time – 10 min ago!' The aromastick anchored this successful relaxation and Deborah used it by herself for future cannulation.

BOX 7.9 Suggestions for cannulation

Do not say or repeatedly think
- Your veins are really poor
- We are going to have problems getting the cannula in
- This is going to be difficult
- Nurse J said she had trouble trying to cannulate you last time
- I am really anxious about doing this
- I can't see any good veins
- This is going to take a few attempts
- This is going to hurt.

Do explain/consider thoughtfully
- View veins as having potential to fully dilate
- Explain how veins can be dilated
- See venous access as an intriguing puzzle to be solved
- Use relaxation and imagery to visualize full dilated veins (both you and the patient)
- Engage in appropriate humour to diffuse the situation
- Use a squeezy ball (Fig. 7.3)
- Explain how the levels of pain and discomfort can be modulated.

Humour and playful language can be useful in stressful situations, this must be sensitively used. For example, the term 'hypnotherapist' is often associated with the entertainment industry, so in introducing ourselves we have often used the 'Little Britain' catch phrase: *'look into my eyes, look into eyes, and don't look around my eyes look into my eyes'* and then clarify the role of 'hypnotherapy' in clinical practice to reassure them that they are in charge at all times.

When using squeezy balls in relaxation training, the balls themselves can be playfully introduced, with the instruction ... *'squeeze really hard!'* Additionally, while using touch therapies or relaxation techniques, it can be playfully suggested that: *'you will become so relaxed that the winning lottery numbers will come flooding into your mind ... I will write them down on a piece of paper'*. Using humour in these ways enacts the 'Law of Dominant Effect', where one strong emotion can supplant another, this concept was first popularized by Coué in 1923 in the book *How to Practice Suggestion and Autosuggestion*.

SUMMARY

There appears to be a bi-directional relationship between coping with distress and life-threatening illness. Loss of control is damaging in stressful situations, where a sense of disempowerment and concerns for the future undermine self-esteem, self-confidence and self-regulation. In acute care situations, it is important for the patient to perceive and experience support, receive helpful information and learn strategies to regain control. The CALM model has been proposed here to guide therapists and health professions. It includes modifying and role modelling language, facilitating grounding through nurturing touch and developing a calming presence. The model emphasizes the engagement of patients in learning about physical signs of anxiety, as well as strategies, which they can choose to employ to regain control and self-regulation.

REFERENCES

Ader, R., 1982. Behaviorally conditioned immunosuppression and murine systemic lupus erythematosus. Science 215, 1534–1536.

Ader, R., Cohen, M., 1975. Behaviorally conditioned immunosuppression. Psychosom. Med. 37, 333–340.

Arias Bal, M.A., Vázquez-Barquero, J.L., Pena, C., et al., 1991. Psychiatric aspects of multiple sclerosis. Acta Psychiatr. Scand. 83, 292–296.

Beecher, H.K., 1955. The powerful placebo. J. Am. Med. Assoc. 159, 1602–1606.

Benson, H., 1996. Timeless healing: the power of biology and belief. Scribner, New York.

Buelow, J.M., 1991. A correlational study of disabilities, stressors and coping methods in victims of multiple sclerosis. J. Neurosurg. Nurs. 23, 247–252.

Choy, Y., Fyer, A.J., Lipsitz, J.D., 2007. Treatment of specific phobia in adults. Clin. Psychol. Rev. 27, 266–286.

Coe, C.L., 1999. Concepts and models of immunological change during prolonged stress. In: Schedlowski, M., Tewes, U. (Eds.), Psychoneuroimmunology: an interdisciplinary introduction. Kluwer Academic/Plenum, New York.

Coué, E., 1923. How to practice suggestion and autosuggestion. American Library Service, New York.

Cox, A.C., Fallowfield, L.J., 2006. After going through chemotherapy I can't see another needle. Eur. J. Oncol. Nurs. 11, 43–48.

Deacon, B., Abramowitz, J., 2006. Fear of needles and vasovagal reactions among phlebotomy patients. Anxiety Disord. 20, 946–960.

Freeman, L.W., 2001. Research on mind-body effects. In: Freeman, L.W., Lawlis, G.F. (Eds.), Complementary & alternative medicine: a research-based approach. Mosby, London.

Glaser, R., Rice, J., Sheridan, J., et al., 1987. Stress related immune suppression: health implications. Brain Behaviour and Immunity 1, 7–20.

Groer, M., Ohnesorge, C., 1993. Menstrual-cycle lengthening and reduction in premenstrual distress through guided imagery. J. Holis. Nurs. 11, 286–294.

Groer, M., Mozingo, J., Droppleman, P., 1994. Measures of salivary immunoglobulin A and state anxiety after a nursing back rub. Appl. Nurs. Res. 7, 2–6.

Henry, J.P., 1986. Neuroendocrine patterns of emotional response. In: Emotion:

theory, research and experiences. Academic Press, San Diego.

Holmes, T.H., Rahe, R.H., 1967. The social readjustment rating scale. J. Psychosom. Res. 11, 213–218.

Iskihan, V., Comez, T., Dames, Z., 2004. Job stress and coping strategies in healthcare professional working with cancer patients. Eur. J. Oncol. 8, 234–244.

Kiecolt-Glaser, J., Garner, W., Speicher, C., et al., 1984. Psychosocial modifiers of immunocompetence in medical students. Psychosom. Med. 46, 7–14.

Lacovides, A., Fountoulakis, K.N., Kaprinsis, S.T., et al., 2000. The relationship between job stress, burnout and clinical depression. J. Affect. Disord. 75, 209–221.

Lazarus, R., Folkman, S., 1984. Stress, appraisal, and coping. Springer, New York.

Lazarus, R., Folkman, S., 1989. Manual for the study of daily hassles and uplifts scales. Consulting Psychologists Press, Palo Alto.

Livneh, H., Antonak, R.F., 1997. Psychosocial adaptation to chronic illness and disability. Aspen, Gaithersburg.

Lloyd, R., 1990. Possible mechanisms of psychoneuroimmunological interactions. In: Ornstein, R., Swencionis, C. (Eds.), The healing brain. Guildford Press, London.

Maycock, P., Mackereth, P., 2009. Helping smokers to stop. International Therapist 86, 18–19.

McCain, N.L., Zeller, J.M., Cella, D.F., et al., 1994. A study of stress management in HIV disease (Abstract). Proceedings of the American Academy of Nursing HIV/AIDS Nursing Care Summit. Washington American Nurse's Association.

Parrish, C.L., Radomsky, A.S., Dugas, M.J., 2008. Anxiety-control strategies: is there room for neutralization in successful exposure treatment? Clin. Psychol. Rev. 28, 1400–1412.

Rabin, B.S., Cohen, S., Ganguli, R., et al., 1989. Bidirectional interaction between the central nervous system and the immune system. Crit. Rev. Immunol. 9, 279–312.

Rotter, 1975. Some problems and misconceptions related to the construct of internal versus external control of reinforcement. J. Consult. Clin. Psychol. 43, 56–67.

Sterling, P., Eyer, J., 1992. Allostasis: a new paradigm to explain arousal pathology. In: Fisher, S., Reason, J. (Eds.), Handbook of life stress, cognition and health. John Wiley, Chichester.

Wolitzky-Taylor, K.B., Horowitz, J.D., Powers, M.B., et al., 2008. Psychological approaches in the treatment of specific phobias: a meta-analysis. Clin. Psychol. Rev. 28, 1021–1037.

FURTHER READING

Buckle, J., 2003. Clinical aromatherapy: essential oils in practice. Churchill Livingstone, London.

Freeman, L.W., Lawlis, G.F. (Eds.), 2001. Complementary & alternative medicine: a research-based approach. Mosby, London.

Kienle, G.S., Kiene, H., 2001. A critical reanalysis of the concept, magnitude and existence of placebo effects. In: Peters, D. (Ed.), Understanding the placebo effect in complementary medicine: theory, practice and research. Churchill Livingstone, London.

Mackereth, P., Carter, A. (Eds.), 2006. Massage & bodywork: adapting therapies for cancer care. Elsevier Science, London.

Mackereth, P., Tiran, D. (Eds.), 2002. Clinical reflexology: a guide for health professionals. Churchill Livingstone, Edinburgh.

Spencer, J.W., 1999. Essential issues in complementary/alternative medicine. In: Spencer, J.W., Jacobs, J.J. (Eds.), Complementary/alternative medicine: an evidence-based approach. Mosby, St Louis.

USEFUL RESOURCES

Journals
The International Journal of Clinical Aromatherapy.

Journal of Essential Oil Therapeutics.

Recognizing and integrating 'hypnotic trance' within touch therapy work

Ann Carter • Peter A. Mackereth

8

CHAPTER CONTENTS

CHAPTER OUTLINE

This chapter explores a range of therapeutic interventions that utilize 'hypnotic trance' to improve well-being and promote resilience in the face of illness or coping with loss. Patients and their carers frequently achieve a trance-like state when receiving complementary therapies which involve touch. In the authors' view, trance can occur independently of a structured hypnotherapy session. This raises a number of issues, in particular safety and the importance of language and aftercare.

© 2010 Elsevier Ltd.
DOI: 10.1016/B978-0-7020-3082-6.00010-1

KEY WORDS

Touch
Trance
Synergistic resource
Boundaries
HEARTS
Emotion
Contracts and safety

INTRODUCTION

The separation between mind and body exists both in medicine and in hypnotherapy practice. Hypnotherapists do not commonly touch patients during trance; a patient receiving hypnotherapy will expect to have an auditory experience where trance is facilitated by the therapist's voice and the skilled use of language. A skilled hypnotherapist will observe and involve the patient's physical responses during treatment, taking cues from the patient's reactions to make adjustments to the therapeutic approach. Patients may become engaged in trance states that facilitate a discharge of feelings, emotional processing and disclosures of concerns and insights. In turn, these may contribute to the patient identifying what s/he may need to move forward, to become more resilient and committed to his/her own well-being.

Practitioners who use therapies which involve touch, such as massage, reflexology and aromatherapy will recognize states of deep relaxation which can be achieved through 'hands-on' work and which may also be recognized as 'trance'. Dependent upon the skills of the therapist to notice physical cues, or to be curious about physical and emotional responses, a patient may be left to work through emerging feelings or recalled memories with variable support. In complementary therapy, the process where emotion is released, during or after the treatment, is often referred to as a 'healing crisis'; the occurrence is usually perceived as temporary and judged beneficial in the longer term (Griffiths 1995, Vickers 1996).

Some of the more common physical signs of deep relaxation and emotional processing are given in Box 8.1. This list is not exhaustive; however, it is likely that these signs will be familiar to most therapists. Therapists may refer to this state as relaxation, day dreaming, reverie, or simply 'chilling out'. It is less likely that therapists will equate the similarities of deep relaxation with hypnotic trance. Most patients enter this state easily without the use of recognized induction techniques or deepeners. There is good argument to assert that all hypnosis is self-hypnosis, a natural 'altered' state into which, given certain conditions, most people will find themselves drifting. Signs of deep relaxation and emotional processing which are comparable with hypnotic trance are given in Box 8.1.

Are trance states facilitated only by a therapist? We need to remember that children (and some adults) become so absorbed by stories that they lose track of time and forget worries and concerns. Being drawn in by a hobby, book, motorway driving or listening to music can cause individuals to enter

> **BOX 8.1 Signs of deep relaxation and emotional processing during touch therapies**
>
> - Conversation slows/ceases
> - Physical relaxation of muscles, twitching, involuntary movements
> - Head droops if sitting, sinks back if lying down
> - Changes in breathing, so it may become deeper and slower
> - Intermittent eye closure
> - Full eye closure
> - Rapid eye movement
> - Change of pallor, e.g. flushing, warming
> - Relaxed jaw
> - Increased salivation
> - Increased peristalsis which may be audible
> - Moist eyes and tear tracking
> - Flatus/burping
> - Yawning/sighing
> - Post-session emotional release, disclosures and insights.

a 'trance' state. The state can cease when it is interrupted by a thought, a noise or a change/cue in the environment.

Having completed hypnotherapy training and advanced bodywork training, the authors recognize that trance states can occur without establishing a formal contract for hypnotic trance. Therapists may recognize when both themselves and the patient have entered a trance state simultaneously. Milne (1995) has referred to trance as a 'glamour' or an expanded state of awareness – 'a larger me'. In this state, bodyworkers typically become more focused, experience heightened awareness and an increased connection to the patient; time distortion can occur for both the patient and therapist. Physical and emotional states can be sensed, which may not be normally noticed when both patient and therapist are in an everyday 'busy' state.

TOUCH: EVIDENCE FOR CHANGE IN MENTAL STATES

The use of touch and the human voice in trance induction is not unusual and can be identified in everyday activities. Stroking and holding babies and children to calm, reassure, promote sleep and provide comfort, all are facets of parental care in both the human and the animal world. Touch therapies alone have been the subject of numerous research studies. Tiffany Field and colleagues (1996) investigated the effects of touch therapies on children. They provided 20 pre-school children with 20 min of massage twice a week for 5 weeks. The treatment group had better behaviour ratings on state vocalization, activity and cooperation after the massage sessions comparing first and last day scores. In a second study by a team (Hart et al 1998), another group of 20 pre-school students received massage with notable changes in cognitive performance for the treatment group. It was identified that massage for children rated as highly strung and anxious, showed greater improvement.

In adults, massage has been found to reduce itching, pain and anxiety in a study by Field et al (2000) with 20 patients with burn injuries. In patients hospitalized for cancer treatment ($n = 41$), Smith et al (2002) investigated effects of massage with 20 compared with an attention-only control group ($n = 21$). Significant changes were reported in the massage group for pain, symptom distress and sleep scores. Notably, the control had a marked deterioration in sleep scores.

HEARTS: A COMBINED APPROACH TO RELAXATION AND TRANCE INDUCTION

Sometimes a patient may find relaxation difficult through the use of the therapist's voice alone and music is often used to aid the process. Similarly, patients experiencing touch therapy may want to 'interact'; depending on the content of the 'talking', the therapy session can become little more than a 'past-time'. However, Carter (2006) developed an approach to facilitate a relaxation for individuals who find a relaxed state difficult to achieve, either through the use of touch or the voice alone. While working with patients who had cancer and their carers, she developed a multifaceted approach where both the skilful use of touch and the sound of the human voice could be intentionally combined to promote relaxation. She describes this combination of interventions as 'holding body and mind', so both can feel relaxed at the same time (Carter 2006). This approach was described as the HEARTS Process; HEARTS being a mnemonic which stands for Hands on, Empathy, Aromas, Relaxation, Textures and Sound. The essence of HEARTS was based on the lines of the poem:

But, Oh, for the touch of the vanished hand and the sound of a voice that is still …

(Tennyson, cited in Autton 1999: 108)

Physical touch is always a constant in HEARTS. The aim is to enable patients to achieve a state of relaxation in the easiest way possible using gentle stroking, holding and varying pressures. If the approaches do not have the desired effect, then the human voice can be introduced to provide very simple diversions for the mind and to reduce the internal 'chatter'. HEARTS is always given through clothes or an additional covering. The textures of the covering, which can include the patient's own clothes, bed clothes, a blanket or a large towel play an important role in the process through utilizing the sensory stimulation of the receptors in the skin. Aromatherapy oils can also be used, although this is only feasible where the therapist is a qualified aromatherapist or where s/he has prescribed the oils for individual patient use.

The effects of this process can be profound (see Box 8.2). In this case study and without consciously realizing it, the therapist had carried out a trance induction using the resources of skilful touch and the human voice.

BODYWORK: CATALYSTS FOR TRANCE

We suggest that there are at least three useful ways in which a bodywork therapist can support a patient through facilitating deep relaxation via touch, which then becomes a trance state.

> **BOX 8.2 Case study 1**
>
> Max, age 35, had been given bad news about his prognosis. He arrived for a half hour 'emergency session' to help him to 'calm down'. Max had been told by the doctor he needed to 'come down off the ceiling' but this was proving impossible. He claimed to have never relaxed in his life, but was going to fight the illness with everything he had. He then gave the therapist the challenge, 'I bet you won't be able to get me to relax either!'
>
> Max remained fully clothed and the therapist covered him with a warm towel. Initially, his hands were clenched; his legs were stiff and his toes pointed towards the ceiling. The therapist then put her hands on Max's head and softly suggested:
>
> *My hands will look after your thoughts ... and for a few moments I invite you to take your attention down to your feet ... become aware of the space between your toes ... and the space between your feet ...*
>
> Still holding Max's head, the therapist then spoke softly to Max's body, reassuring the different parts that they could relax as they did not need to do any work right now. Max's eyes closed within seconds, and within minutes, his breathing became deeper, his legs, feet and hands relaxed and he calmed.

First, the development of rapport between patient and therapist is essential to facilitating an altered state of consciousness. Catalysts for rapport can include mirroring, effective listening, and patient expectations combined with the intentions of the therapist to create a safe and comfortable environment (Fig. 8.1). These and other factors help co-create a sense of safe attachment (see Ch. 5) which allows the patient to move into a hypnotic state.

Second, therapists may have developed resourceful language and presence which engage a patient in positively working with his/her emotional and physical state. This can also include the integrated use of creative imagery, discussed later in this chapter.

Third, therapists routinely work towards creating a nurturing experience, which they reinforce with anchoring through the therapeutic use of touch and supportive language. At the close of the session and beyond, the patient can access a memory of being comforted, feeling restored and more at ease with his/her concerns.

These three processes contribute to engaging the patient in trance, thus enhancing the patient's therapeutic process and reinforcing 'remembered wellness'. This term was coined by Benson (1996) to describe evoked memories of being nurtured, originally ascribed to feeling connected to maternal attachment. All three elements become a synergistic resource for the patient in 'living well', despite challenges and concerns. This is illustrated by all four case studies in this chapter.

INTEGRATING CREATIVE IMAGERY IN BODYWORK

Creative imagery can be an invaluable tool when used in combination with touch therapies. Examples of this practice have been reported in reflexology, craniosacral and other psychodynamic forms of bodywork (Hodkinson

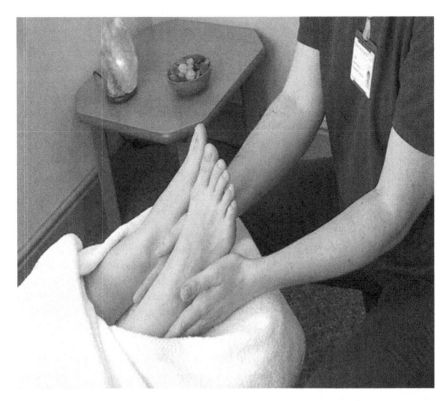

FIG 8.1 Holding the feet – holding the person.

et al 2006, Staunton 2002). Creative imagery and creative visualization are often used to describe similar practices. However, in practice, they can be distinguished. Visualization suggests the use of one sense only, that which can be seen. In this chapter, the term 'imagery' is used to describe a multi-sensory experience, with the visual, auditory, kinaesthetic and olfactory senses blended in various combinations to create 'the journey'. The gustatory or taste sense can also be included to stimulate salivary flow, but is most useful in specific situations (see Ch. 7).

Creative imagery may be a therapist-led technique where the patient is guided where to go, what to experience and make the return. This method of delivery is usually dependent on a prepared or rehearsed script. Common examples are a walk in the country, a beach, or a garden. A more person-centred approach can enable an individual to travel to a place where s/he would like to be, then to explore the surroundings in terms of sensory experience and bring back a feeling, word or imagined object useful to him/her in the present. When this approach is used, the patient provides the content, which can be very helpful as it puts him/her in control of the process. A variation on this approach is for the therapist to discuss the patient's 'preferred content' before the session starts, and then to co-create a 'journey' which contains the patient's suggested content. The patient can give feedback and refine his/her own 'journey' for use in subsequent sessions or independently at home.

BOX 8.3 Case study 2

Tricia, aged 52, was very concerned about having a procedure for draining ascites (fluid) from her abdomen. She had received massage on several occasions and she found it pleasant and relaxing. She voiced her concerns to the therapist who said he would use an 'easy to learn' technique which Tricia could access before and during the procedure. Towards the end of the massage, the therapist suggested to Tricia that she could quickly recall:

... how relaxed you are now ... and how good it felt to receive the massage ... my hands and voice guiding you to a deeper state of relaxation ... this thought will enable your mind to drift back to how relaxed you are feeling right now ... knowing that the procedure will bring comfort and make your breathing easier.

Before having the procedure, Tricia asked if she could have a few moments to 'get herself relaxed'. She remembered her experience with massage and was able to complete the procedure without difficulty.

INCORPORATING 'REMEMBERED WELLNESS'

Utilizing the concept of 'remembered wellness' within bodywork practice invites the patient to embed the experience of receiving relaxing touch. Patients can also learn to access this remembered experience when wanting to rest or fall asleep. The therapist can also suggest that the treatment experience can be revisited when the patient finds medical or procedural interventions particularly challenging. A case study which illustrates the use of suggestion is described in Box 8.3. Some further suggestions for 'anchoring' pleasant touch therapy experiences as support for aftercare can include:

... noticing the support, being held ... notice how relaxed you feel ... and at any time you can recall the experience your body remembers .... and know that you can go back to a place of calm, recharge your batteries – you practice this at home ... you will sleep more deeply and awaken more refreshed ... as you breathe out in your sleep your body will release tension ... you will sleep easier and awake refreshed ...

THE IMPORTANCE OF USING RESOURCEFUL LANGUAGE

The power of the language a therapist uses cannot be overestimated in interactions with patients. Rushworth (1999: 40–41) describes a situation where a group of male patients were watching a football match; they were totally absorbed in the game, making jovial comments and generally enjoying the football. Then a nurse asked the patients if they wanted 'something for the pain'. The mood suddenly changed as the patients were reminded of pain and discomfort, the joviality subsided, and the group became quieter.

Rushworth (1999) suggests that it would have been more resourceful to ask, 'Is everyone comfortable?' and her words would have suggested 'comfort' and reinforced the group's state of ease. Rushworth also suggests that the words 'comfort boost' could be more resourceful than 'pain killer'.

HOW CAN THE TOUCH THERAPIST UTILIZE THE TRANCE STATE?

Utilizing hypnotherapy techniques within a touch therapy, such as massage, aromatherapy and reflexology is not commonly reported, but may be practised informally. In some therapies, such as craniosacral therapy and psychodynamic bodywork, processing information given in trance is a recognized part of the therapy (Staunton 2002, Upledger 2003). A touch therapist who is also a trained hypnotherapist may want to combine the two approaches for 'change work' or to enhance the treatment. This additional component must be contracted for with the patient. Alternatively, a hypnotherapist and touch therapist can work with a patient together, using both modalities in tandem. This dual approach requires planning and collaboration, with both therapists communicating verbally and non-verbally to ensure safety and shared purpose. The degree of involvement of both therapists will depend on the patient's goals for the session. For example, when working with a patient's phobia, the hypnotherapist would 'lead' the session, the bodywork therapist providing gentle nurturing touch, which may require subtle direction (see Case study 3, Box 8.4).

EMOTIONAL RELEASE AND SAFE THERAPEUTIC PRACTICE

A patient's experience of touch-induced trance may lead to a release of emotions. Sometimes, the patient may spontaneously enter a state of regression, where involuntary movements spontaneously occur. The legs and arms are frequently involved; sometimes the individual will turn on to his/her side and adopt a fetal position. Alternatively, s/he may adopt a physical position associated with the 'incident' which occurred at an earlier time (Upledger

---

BOX 8.4 Case study 3

Janice, aged 51, had attended a reflexology session prior to chemotherapy. Janice found herself becoming anxious the day before her hospital appointment, resorting to asking for a sedative to get through the cannulation. Wanting to avoid becoming dependent on medication, Janice requested help from her therapist. Noticing that Janice was in a tearful and distracted state, the reflexologist enlisted the assistance of a hypnotherapist.

On meeting Janice, the hypnotherapist noticed how anxious and withdrawn she was, almost as if she was afraid to breathe deeply. As the hypnotherapist gently worked with relaxation techniques and the reflexologist held Janice's feet she noticed that Janet seemed to drift. Followed by a series of deep breaths, tears started to flow down Janice's cheeks. The hypnotherapist asked, 'What has come into your thoughts?' Janice said, 'When I was just eight I was left alone in hospital and I was really frightened ... I didn't know where my mum had gone.' Acknowledging this trauma the hypnotherapist asked, 'What do you need from us right now?' Janice said 'Please carry on ... I don't really need the medication .... I feel very safe just now.' Janice was able to use the relaxation techniques at home (supported by a CD). She reported that she slept well that night and had no further problems with cannulation.

1990). Without prior knowledge of trance states and the possible occurrence of emotional release/regression, the therapist is placed in a challenging position, questioning how s/he can best respond and help the patient.

For those skilled in body psychotherapy or craniosacral work, it would be appropriate to consider stopping or 'stilling' the touch – the therapist may want to ask the individual, 'What is happening for you?' and 'What do you need from me right now?' These questions are an intervention and require the therapist to be able to work in a skilled, reflective and dynamic way. Using this approach in touch and bodywork therapies requires additional training and ongoing supervision (Mackereth & Carter 2006a).

It is essential that therapists are aware of their own bodies and physical responses when working with patients. On a practical level this means considering health and safety issues to develop strategies to avoid strain or injury (Pyves & Mackereth 2002). These can include ensuring ergonomic movements, appropriate use and positioning of equipment (couch/bed height), careful and supported postural changes and avoiding lifting and repetitive movements.

Traditionally, in hypnotherapy, psychotherapy and counselling work, touch has been an activity to be carefully considered and often avoided. In part, this separation of body and mind has been thought to safeguard the work, but Mackereth and Carter (2006b) have suggested that this may be primarily for the therapist's protection rather than the safety of the patient. Therapists have started to recognize that their own bodies and reactions are important to therapeutic work. For example, therapists working with patients may become aware of a deep heaviness (feeling sleepy or weighted down) in their own bodies, or a rising level of anxiety (e.g. changes in breathing, swallowing more frequently, etc.). This has been termed 'somatic countertransference' and is well recognized in the body psychotherapy literature (Shaw 2003). This phenomenon may be the therapists' shift in awareness of their own bodies, triggered by engaging mindfully with another person and his/her body. It could also be due to working at some level of intuition related to changes in the patient's affective/emotional state during treatment (see Case study 4, Box 8.5).

BOX 8.5 Case study 4

Angela, aged 36, a carer for her mother with ovarian cancer, had been feeling very overwhelmed by the role and with thoughts of losing her. At the beginning of a one-to-one session, Angela agreed to use a guided journey to a beach as the basis of a creative imagery session. The therapist guided her arrival to the beach and suggested she dip her toes in the water, but then noticed Angela becoming agitated. The therapist did not feel comfortable either and so stopped the session. Asking how she was, Angela reported feeling anxious after remembering an early near-drowning experience as a child. The therapist acknowledged the fear and her survival. In talking more, Angela shared that her mother had encouraged her to get back into the water and she had become a very good swimmer. Angela talked about how proud she was of her mother and how she had helped her to overcome fear.

In the next sessions having had supervision, the therapist reminded Angela that she could indicate if she wanted to stop the session at any point. This reinforcement of the contract was included given the insight gained from the first session.

BOUNDARIES OF PRACTICE ISSUES

It is important that the therapist is able to explain clearly and confidently the benefits of using trance to enhance the proposed body treatment. Some patients may be fearful of 'hypnotherapy' but will consent to the inclusion of imagery techniques so long as formal induction techniques and deepeners are not used. It is important to be clear what consent is and whether a patient is competent to give it. Some bodywork therapists may not be enthusiastic about introducing creative imagery into their practice. Hypnotherapists and bodywork therapists working together can provide opportunities for learning, recognizing trance, and feeling safe and even more confident in integrating creative imagery. It is important to realize that the therapist may have a limited knowledge of a patient's history in terms of physical or psychological abuse, which may make it painful or distressing for the patient to participate. Illness or surgery may also alter how a patient may perceive themselves physically, which can lead to withdrawal and embarrassment, when he/she has to relate to individuals in new situations. This can make it difficult for individuals to feel comfortable participating and engaging in what might be a new experience, either in a creative imagery session on a one to one basis or in a group. The section that follows examines these issues in relation to safe and appropriate practice.

PREPARATORY QUESTIONS FOR ALL FORMS OF 'RELAXATION' PRACTICE

It is important to acknowledge that the following guidance relates to therapies which involve any form of creative imagery and relaxation work. Additionally, therapists may also be using progressive muscle relaxation training (see Ch. 6). From working in clinical settings, we have developed a series of questions adapted from work by Campbell et al (2006); the list below is intended as a guide, rather than being prescriptive or exhaustive.

Questions for the touch therapist and/or hypnotherapist

- Will the use of a hypnotherapy intervention contribute to the overall goal of the session?
- Is the therapist(s) able to explain clearly and concisely the rationale for including hypnosis in a bodywork treatment?
- If working alone, does the therapist have the hypnotherapy skills to work safely and effectively with patients at an emotional level during and after the treatment?
- Does the therapist have the managerial support necessary to work with a patient?
- Is sufficient space and time available conducive to the intervention proposed?
- How comfortable is the therapist about asking the patient for feedback or stopping to clarify the work at any time?
- Is the therapist calm and sufficiently centred to be present for this person?

- Does the therapist know to whom a referral can be made if more in-depth work is required?
- Is there an experienced person with hypnotherapy training to provide supervision on an ongoing basis?

Questions for the carer/patient/staff

- Does the patient want to be involved in hypnosis as well as touch therapy?
- Is s/he competent, able and willing to consent to the intervention?
- Does s/he understand the therapist's level of skill and the boundaries of this approach to the work?
- Are there any impediments to using hypnosis with the patient?
- Has the patient been asked about factors which may influence the approach to the hypnosis?
- Have arrangements been made with the patient/carer to follow-up the session, and to provide a means of contact or support, should it be needed?

CONTRACTING

An initial contract for any therapeutic intervention is essential, not only in empowering the patient/carer in making choices and decisions, but also in clarifying the purpose of treatment and setting realistic goals. Contracts are open to renegotiation as treatments progress and may be changed in subsequent sessions. For example, a patient, may initially want just reflexology, but may later raise an issue where worries and concerns surface just when he/she is trying to fall asleep.

THE IMPORTANCE OF SAYING 'NO'

It is often too easy to invite a patient or carer to take part in hypnosis as well as 'hands on' therapy, without considering that this might be a very unusual activity for them. A therapist's intention to be even more effective by offering more than one approach at the same time, may be experienced as 'too much' by the patient, or he/she may wonder why s/he may need more than one treatment. To please the therapist, a patient may feel s/he must go along with whatever is offered. Sometimes people can be overwhelmed by the illness. Carers may be overwhelmed by fears for their loved one. Mackereth (2000) argues that some patients may be compliant with healthcare professionals' requests to avoid being judged as demanding or difficult and risk compromising care. Acquiescing can be easier than saying, 'No, I don't want this right now.' It is therefore essential that while 9 out of 10 people will willingly take part, therapists may need to recognize and support the patient's right to decline.

Agreeing that a patient can ask to stop the session and clarify the contract at any time could be tested at the start of the first session. For example, a therapist could suggest that the patient actually stops the session verbally in the first few minutes and then ask for a change in the work. Just stopping for a moment at the patient's request can help affirm the contract agreement and give the patient confidence for some change in the approach or to stop the session. Hunter and Struve (1998) recommend that therapists protect themselves and their clients by having a clear contract and consent for any therapeutic work. An important principle with any work is that patients are supported and encouraged to create their own way of relaxing or journeying with imagery. Monitoring is about the ability and sensitivity of a therapist to notice responses to the therapeutic work, both from the patient and in themselves as the therapy proceeds. For example, 'Is the patient breathing more slowly and deeply?' 'How relaxed am I?' 'Am I entering trance state with the patient?' The case study in Box 8.5 demonstrates the need to be vigilant.

Below is a summary of the practical considerations when preparing an individual therapy session:

- Ensure that the patient/carer has consented for the intervention and knows that they can ask for the session to stop at any point
- Assess whether the patient/carer can sit or lie comfortably for the 15–30 min and limit the session time to a maximum of 30 min
- Evaluate treatment sessions with the patient (or carer) and maintain confidential documentation
- Be aware that a patient may be unable to consent, e.g. is he/she confused or disorientated? Have they imbued alcohol, taken sedatives, strong narcotics or non-prescribed substances? If ability to consent is in doubt it is professional practice to not treat someone, no matter who has referred them.
- Does the patient have a raised temperature or is he/she feeling unwell/breathless?
- Seek advice from the referrer if asked to provide creative imagery to an individual with a history of mental health problems.

SUMMARY

We have argued here that touch therapies and relaxation techniques can trigger trance-like states in patients who are vulnerable, experiencing a major life crisis and whose bodies and minds are open to the processes. Achieving a trance state through touch and relaxation may be influenced by the therapist's compassion, skilled presence and curiosity. It is important to consider safety issues, skill level and supervision requirements of therapists combining hypnotherapy with bodywork. Being vigilant and knowing boundaries are important. Our reflections in developing this chapter lead us to recommend that hypnotherapists consider working with touch therapists in the interest of patients. What integrative hypnotherapy teaches us is the importance of connecting mind and body through language and touch. We have been privileged to assist and support touch therapists to learn more about hypnotherapy and we hope this chapter will encourage hypnotherapists to learn more about touch.

Autton, N., 1999. Touch: an exploration. Darton, Longman & Todd, London.

Benson, H., 1996. Timeless healing: the power of biology and belief. Scribner, New York.

Campbell, G., Mackereth, P.A., Sylt, P., 2006. Adapting chair massage for carers, staff and patients. In: Mackereth, P., Carter, A. (Eds.), Massage & bodywork: adapting therapies in cancer care. Elsevier Science, London.

Carter, A., 2006. HEARTS. In: Mackereth, P., Carter, A. (Eds.), Massage & bodywork: adapting therapies in cancer care. Elsevier Science, London.

Field, T., Kilmer, T., Hernandez-Reif, M., et al., 1996. Preschool children's sleep and wake behaviour: effects of massage therapy. Early Child Development and Care 120, 39–44.

Field, T., Peck, M., Hernandez-Reif, M., et al., 2000. Post burn itching, pain and psychological symptoms are reduced with massage therapy. J. Burn Care Rehabil. 21, 189–193.

Griffiths, P., 1995. Reflexology. In: Rankin-Box, D. (Ed.), The nurse's handbook of complementary therapies. Churchill Livingstone, London.

Hart, S., Field, T., Hernandez-Reif, M., et al., 1998. Preschoolers' cognitive performance improves following massage. Early Child Development and Care 143, 59–64.

Hodkinson, E., Cook, B., Mackereth, P., 2006. Mackereth, P., Carter, A. (Eds.), Massage & bodywork: adapting therapies in cancer care. Elsevier Science, London.

Hunter, M., Struve, J., 1998. The ethical use of touch in psychotherapy. Sage, London.

Mackereth, P., 2000. Tough places to be tender: contracting for happy or 'good enough' endings in therapeutic massage/ bodywork? Complementary Therapies in Nursing and Midwifery 6 (3), 11–115.

Mackereth, P., Carter, A. (Eds.), 2006a. Massage & bodywork: adapting therapies in cancer care. Elsevier Science, London.

Mackereth, P., Carter, A., 2006b. Nurturing resilience: touch therapies in palliative care. Journal of Holistic Healthcare 3 (1), 24–28.

Milne, H., 1995. The heart of listening: a visionary approach to craniosacral work. North Atlantic Books, Berkeley.

Pyves, G., Mackereth, P., 2002. Practising safely and effectively: introducing the 'no-hands' approach, a paradigm shift in the theory and practice of reflexology. In: Mackereth, D., Tiran, D. (Eds.), Clinical reflexology: a guide for health professionals. Churchill Livingstone, Edinburgh.

Rushworth, C., 1999. Making a difference in cancer care: practical techniques in palliative and curative treatment, second ed. Souvenir Press, London.

Shaw, R., 2003. The embodied psychotherapist: the therapist's body story. Brunner-Routledge, Hove, Sussex.

Smith, M.C., Kemp, J., Hemphill, L., et al., 2002. Outcomes for therapeutic massage for hospitalized cancer patients. J. Nurs. Scholarsh. 34 (3), 257–262.

Staunton, T., 2002. Body psychotherapy (advancing theory in therapy). Brunner-Routledge, Hove, Sussex.

Upledger, J., 1990. Somato-emotional release and beyond. UI Publishing, Florida.

Upledger, J., 2003. Cell talk – talking to your cell(f). North Atlantic Books, Berkeley.

Vickers, A., 1996. Massage and aromatherapy: a guide for health professionals. Chapman & Hall, London.

FURTHER READING

Battino, R., 2000. Guided imagery and other approaches to healing. Crown House, Carmarthen.

Freeman, L.W., 2001. Research on mind-body effects. In: Freeman, L.W., Lawlis, G.F. (Eds.), Mosby's complementary & alternative medicine: a research-based approach. Mosby, London.

Mackereth, P., Carter, A. (Eds.), 2006. Massage & bodywork: adapting therapies in cancer care. Elsevier Science, London.

Recognizing and integrating 'hypnotic trance' within touch therapy work

McFarland, D., 2000. Body secrets. Healing Arts Press, Los Angeles.

Montagu, A., 1986. Touching: the human significance of the skin. Harper and Row, London.

Pert, C., 1997. Molecules of emotion. Simon and Shuster, Sydney.

Rubenfeld, I., 2000. The listening hand: how to combine bodywork and psychotherapy to heal emotional pain. Piatkus, London.

USEFUL RESOURCE

Touch Research Institute, Miami, USA, www.miami.edu/touch-research.

Body image, sexuality, weight loss and hypnotherapy

Anne Cawthorn • Kathy Stephenson

9

CHAPTER CONTENTS

CHAPTER OUTLINE

This chapter explores issues relating to body image, sexuality and weight issues. It considers how these affect the individual during health, illness, accident and following sexual abuse. Different assessment models are explored alongside a number of hypnotherapeutic approaches which are applicable in this area of practice. A number of case studies illustrate how these apply in practice and include working with patient's dreams.

© 2010 Elsevier Ltd.
DOI: 10.1016/B978-0-7020-3082-6.00011-3

KEY WORDS

Body image
Sexuality
Weight
DIRECT model
Self-esteem
Self-worth
Dreams

INTRODUCTION

Problems associated with people's sense of their own body have increased over recent years and discussions about body image are much more commonly found in the media, alongside those within health and social care. Orbach (2009: 1) suggests that 'millions struggle on a daily basis against troubled and shaming feelings about the way their bodies appear'. Societal obsession with the perfect body, which includes being beautiful, fit, and slim and remaining youthful; all exert unrealistic pressures on individuals. The images of perfection are everywhere and our bodies are being shaped by forces beyond our control (Orbach 2009). It is not hard to see therefore why society is beginning to acknowledge this as a growing problem.

Over recent years, an increasing amount of literature has emerged, with a number of authors attempting to define body image and develop models relating to practice. Grogan (1999) defined body image as a person's perceptions, thoughts and feelings about his or her body, which incorporates appearance, body size, shape and attractiveness. Concern about our bodies is normal and allows us to have healthy body awareness. However, excessive bodily concern can lead on to an abnormal focus and can result in bodily obsession or body dysmorphic disorder (Webster's Dictionary 2008).

A broader view of body image would include more than just the issues relating to appearance but would involve the psychological perception by the individual of their body as being intact, whole and properly functioning. There are many life-threatening and life-limiting illnesses which can cause body image changes, or which impact on how the body functions; these include strokes, multiple sclerosis, rheumatoid arthritis, diabetes and cancer, to name but a few. In addition, the result of life-changing events such as accidents, surgery including amputations and colostomies, leave many people with body image issues. Some of these changes are temporary, while many remain permanent and require the person to adjust to them.

Disfigurement is a particularly difficult body image problem relating to more than just the visual effect of the disfigurement, but linking with the patient's thoughts and feelings about how it was acquired. Barraclough (1999) reminds us that people cope differently with disfigurement and suggests that some people can be very self-conscious to changes that are not immediately obvious to others. It is important therefore, to assess the patient's perception of the problem, while suspending our own judgement. One way of doing this is to adopt an approach developed by Berne's (1972) and 'think Martian'.

When asking the person to describe how they see the problem, we suspend our personal knowledge base and judgement, in an effort to see it through their eyes. This technique is very powerful because, in addition to being empathetic, the therapist also enters into the patient's 'frame of reference' by listening to the language and metaphors they use to describe themselves.

Body image is closely aligned with a person's sexuality and as such, the authors recommend a broader working definition in order that all aspects of the patient's persona are acknowledged. White (2006) takes a holistic view in relation to this area of practice suggesting that:

Sexuality embraces the associated concepts of sexual identity, sexual expression or behaviour and intimacy. It is also closely allied with concepts such as body image or self concept, gender identity, gender roles and relationships

White (2006: 676)

Freud (1936) also recommended a similarly broad approach, reminding therapists that sex is something we do but sexuality is something we are and as such incorporates many facets of the individual. It is important therefore, that when assessing patients, prior to offering hypnotherapy techniques, we need to ascertain how their body image concerns relate to the broader view they have of themselves, and whether this affects their roles and relationships with others.

ASSESSMENT MODELS

Assessment of body image and sexual concerns is dependent on the therapist's attitude, knowledge base and skills in eliciting the patient's perception of their problems. Three models which provide a framework to assist this process will be considered.

DIRECT/NEGOTIATION MODEL

The DIRECT/Negotiation Model (Box 9.1) utilizes a staged approach to assessing body image and sexual concerns which allows the therapist and patient to proceed at a mutually agreed level. It is a 6-stage approach which is particularly useful when negotiating with the patient as to whether they wish to discuss and work with particularly sensitive areas. Negotiation is

---

BOX 9.1 The DIRECT/Negotiation model: a 6-stage approach to assessment

1. **D**evelop the relationship/*Negotiate before moving on*
2. **I**nvite the person to tell you about themselves and inquire how any body image concerns impact on them as an individual/*Negotiate*
3. **R**eflect back your willingness to hear their concerns/*Negotiate*
4. **E**licit and **E**xplore their concerns/*Negotiate*
5. **C**ommunicate your understanding of their problem/*Negotiate how these might be resolved*
6. **T**reatment/**T**herapy can be *negotiated* and suggestions made to how hypnotherapy techniques can help in resolving their concerns.

used to elicit what the patient is comfortable working with and is used throughout the assessment, enabling the therapist to proceed at the patient's pace. This can relate to either the depth of communication they are comfortable with, or when negotiating which hypnotherapy approaches they are happy to engage in. (For further explanation of this model, see Chapter 5, and a full version, which also includes Annon's (1976) P.LI.SS.IT (1976) Assessment Model, can be found at: www://learnzone.macmillan.org.uk.)

BODY IMAGE MODEL (PRICE)

Price (1990) developed a 3-stage model which enables the therapist or healthcare professional (HCP) to identify and explore different aspects of a patient's body image:

1. The first aspect is 'body reality'. This is the 'warts and all' of our body image which we may or may not choose to share with others. Under normal circumstances, the 'body reality' may not be problematic. However, when people are unable to keep these aspects hidden, either due to illness or lack of privacy, problems may begin to emerge. Our body reality changes throughout our lives, with a number of changes occurring at times of transition, such as puberty and menopause. Most people adjust to these changes without any support. However, for some, this can be the time when body image concerns begin to develop. The changes and challenges which occur throughout puberty can be the catalyst for problems such as anorexia and bulimia. Also the losses which occur around and following the menopause, may for some people be more difficult to adjust to.
2. The second aspect of the model is the 'body ideal'. This is the picture in our heads of how we would like to be and may well be unachievable for most people. The media presents the 'ideal look' encouraging us to aim for perfection by promoting youthfulness and vitality. Most people, even the young and beautiful struggle with this ideal and those with body image changes due to illness or injury are often moving further away from the original ideal image they had of themselves. Orbach (2009) questions why bodily contentment is so hard to find and it would appear that the answer might lie in the constant striving for the 'body ideal'.
3. The third aspect of the model is 'body presentation'. This is how we present ourselves to the world and links with the term 'being presentable'. Even this can be greatly compromised when people are ill or taking medication whose side-effects impact on their body image. In these situations, what is often presented to the world, is their body reality (and perhaps a new even less positive body reality), which for some patients is very distressing. Examples might include: hair loss or weight gain from steroids, or where a disfigurement is impossible to hide.

BODY IMAGE MODEL (CASH & PRUZINSKY)

Cash & Pruzinsky (2002) have developed a useful framework for assessing body image concerns. Their book offers a variety of tools which patients can use individually or can be used to form part of their therapy. A body image diary is used as a way of reflecting on their body image concerns. Patients are encouraged to notice:

- Activators – triggering events/situations which raise body image concerns
- Beliefs – what thoughts and interpretations they deduct from this
- Consequences – the emotional tide occurring as a result of the body image concerns being activated.

They are asked to name and record the types of emotions they feel, their intensity (scoring them from 1–10), their duration and any effects they have on their behaviour. This may include avoidance behaviour, which is common in this group. This information can then be used to form the basis of any work undertaken using hypnotherapy.

Applying hypnotherapy

When looking at using hypnotherapy in this area of practice, the following examples may be of use to practitioners.

The American Society for Clinical Hypnosis (2009) suggests three main ways of practicing hypnotherapy:

1. The first is to encourage the use of imagination. Patients are asked to imagine what they see and the therapist may go on to work in a way that helps them to change a negative image. This will be further explored when looking at Cunningham's (2000) model below.
2. The second way is to present ideas or suggestions to the patient, which in the case of body image will help them to use positive suggestions in order to reframe their perception of the problem.
3. The third way is to use hypnotherapy for unconscious exploration and is used to explore motivation or links with past events. Hypnosis avoids the critical censor of the conscious mind, allowing the interface between the conscious and unconscious, which results in the client having the information they need to make the changes.

IMAGERY

Imagery is an important aspect of working with body image issues. Two modes of imagery, which are useful in facilitating this process, are: 'diagnostic' and 'therapeutic' (Cunningham 2000).

Diagnostic imagery

Diagnostic imagery can be used just to elicit information, or in addition can form the basis from which the therapist works using hypnotherapy techniques. During the imagery, ideas/information from the unconscious become available, which is not always accessible from the rational mind. The wealth of information that the unconscious holds, allows patients to gain new information in order to bring about healing. The therapist is the privileged facilitator of this.

Therapeutic imagery

Therapeutic imagery entails working in a positive way with the images the patient presents, based on the principle that images affect body function. The therapist encourages the patient to imagine beneficial changes in the images they see. The patient gets in touch with both their conscious and unconscious, to consult with their 'Inner Healer' in the imagination, to bring about healing from within (Cunningham 2000). From practical experience, patients work well using this approach. They are usually very inventive and can fill up empty spaces with 'magic healing fluid', making it the colour and consistency which is just right for them. They can change parts of the body which look dark and diseased by flushing out all the dark colours and replacing them with bright healing colours. Often the healing comes about in the patient's unconscious through seeing themselves whole again; even though the physical reality may be different.

CLEAN LANGUAGE MODEL

Finally, another useful framework worth consideration is that developed by Grove and Panzer (1991) to resolve traumatic memories. The basis of the model is the use of what they refer to as clean language (using the patient's words). They assert that this ensures that the patient's meaning and resonance remains wholly intact, and is uncontaminated by the therapist's words. Working in this way opens the door to change through developing a much more naturalistic trance which avoids evoking resistance. The therapy begins by inviting the patient to tell their narrative, paying attention to the language they use. This is done by examining the auditory, visual and kinaesthetic channels used, in addition to noting how they use language in order to describe their experiences and inner realities.

The model suggests that a patient may express their internal reality in one of four languages. These are expressed as: memories, symbols, metaphors and semantics, and the therapist's role is to discover which of these appears to be predominant.

Memories

Patients generally recall events from the past. However, Grove and Panzer suggest that memories can also be anticipatory and relate to future events. The memories disclosed can either be real or imagined. They suggest that when working in this dimension the focus should be on the memory, as the words patients use simply give information. It is the memory itself which is the most significant aspect in relation to the therapy which follows (see Case study 1, Box 9.2).

Symbols

In this model, the symbols are internal symbols and differ from Jungian symbols in that they are idiosyncratic rather than being universal symbols. They are located in the body and patients refer to them in terms of physiology such as a 'knot in their stomach'. The therapist's role is to find out what

BOX 9.2 Case study 1

An example from personal practice of working in this way is with Katherine, a 19-year-old girl who had suffered from trichotillomania (hair pulling). She had begun pulling large chunks of her hair out at aged 12 and was still currently doing it. The loss of hair affected her body image and she was anxious to resolve this through hypnotherapy. In therapy, she was encouraged to tell her narrative from the time the hair pulling started. Clean language was used throughout the work with her. When she entered into a conversational trance, memories were her predominant language. We worked with the memories evoked from that time. This involved her witnessing her parent's constant arguments. Not wanting to take sides as she loved each one equally, she described herself as a passive bystander. As she was recalling this, she saw herself as being very isolated, with no one to comfort her. While in trance, she was encouraged to use her adult resources to give (young) Katherine the comfort she needed at that time. This worked well for her and after two sessions, she stopped pulling her hair out.

The healing for Katherine lay in working with her memories. As an adult she was able to provide the support she needed (to young Katherine) in order to soothe her scare, as she witnessed her parents arguments escalating.

the patient feels about the knot rather than focussing on the words used. One particular patient referred to her cancer as 'insidiously strangling her' and the importance of the therapy was to find out what her feelings were in relation to this and to use hypnotherapy to change these feelings.

Metaphors

Metaphors are one way of describing something else and are derived from the patient's experience. They are external to the body. Examples might include having a 'wall between themselves and others', having a 'cloud hanging over them' or describing the illness or its treatments like 'being at the fairground' and being put on new and scary rides. For the therapist, what is visualized is important to work with, e.g. how the patient sees the wall, the cloud, or the fairground rides; their shapes, size, colour, etc. While in trance the therapist can work with these images facilitating the patient to make the changes which are right for them. This may mean removing the brick wall, changing or removing the clouds and converting the fairground scene. The principle is to work with the patient's agenda in helping them to regain their sense of control and security.

Semantics

Semantics is the fourth language and the significance here lies in the private definition of the words for the patient. In semantics, it is the words and not the meanings that have the most important effects. Words like 'burning', 'distressing', 'gutted', 'laid bare', all have private meanings and as therapists, we should never presume to understand their meanings. It is the patient who will guide us to this discovery.

Grove and Panzer (1991) link this way of working with neuro-linguistic programming (NLP) and Ericksonian therapy, in that the therapist matches and paces the patient's language and mirrors their body language. They assert that their model goes further as the adoption of clean language and the structuring of questions, facilitates the patient to naturally go into trance. They describe this as conversational trance, and feel that the benefits arise because patients can go inside to get the information they need, and then give feedback to the therapist in relation to what they see and how they want to work. It also allows the patient to give feedback when they have completed their task.

HYPNOTHERAPY FOR WEIGHT CONTROL

Hypnotherapy can be a very useful tool dealing with weight control issues. It can be used to help clients to re-programme their unconscious attitude to food and also to place less importance to food in relation to their feelings of well-being. Hypnotherapeutic suggestions can be used to increase the appeal of healthy foods and enhance the sensory experience of eating. It is also a useful tool to help to reduce negative self-image and boost positive body image.

During the initial consultation, it is useful to help the client to set a well-formed outcome. A key factor for clients in reaching their desired weight is to have a clear and realistic goal in mind. Focus on what they want, not what they don't want. 'I want to be slim, fit and healthy', rather than 'I don't want to be fat'. This should be specific, e.g. 'I want to lose 1 stone in 2 months' or 'I want to feel comfortable in size 12 clothes'. Visualizing is also key here, and it is useful to help the client develop a clear picture of themselves the way they want themselves to be, 'see yourself looking fit, slim and healthy, make the picture as bright and you can.' This point is reinforced frequently during the hypnotherapy session, as it is important for the client to focus upon how they want to be; to send messages to their unconscious mind to explore every opportunity possible to move towards their goal. Visualization techniques can be a very useful tool in helping the client to develop a positive body image. During hypnosis, the client bypasses critical consciousness and therefore is often able to create a very vivid picture of themselves looking and feeling slim and healthy.

A particularly detrimental aspect of dieting is the obsessive behaviour which is created. When a certain food is 'forbidden' we tend to want to eat it all the more. The restriction of certain foods sets up obsessive behaviour patterns. Strict dieting regimes are antisocial, impossible to maintain long term and lead to yo-yo dieting and low self-esteem. It is important to emphasize that if they want to gain control of their eating patterns, they should not deny themselves any types of food. The aim is to move away from relying on the willpower it takes to follow other people's rules and to move towards listening to their own body. Hypnosis can be used in a way which puts the client in control of their own eating patterns. The following technique is a method of helping the client to tune in to their body's needs.

A significant step to becoming permanently slimmer is to tune into your own personal hunger gauge. This is a highly effective tool to help you become aware of your own body's needs. Imagine a horizontal scale in your stomach marked incrementally with 1 at the bottom up to 10 at the top. One representing a feeling of starvation and physically faint and 10 representing feeling stuffed and nauseous. The points in between range from 2 – very hungry; 3 and 4 – averagely hungry; 5 – neutral; 6 and 7 – nicely satisfied and 8 – quite full. Picture and tune into this gauge whenever you go to eat something, if it registers 5 or above you soon become aware that your body does not need the food. You are always in control with this method, there is no should or shouldn't, just you making your own choices.

Stephenson (2005)

The above technique is often unconsciously used by naturally slim people who also check how their stomach feels when they approach meal times. They often imagine how the food would feel in their stomach over time if they ate it. The thought of sickly sweet fattening food slowly digesting may not be very appealing. Hypnotherapeutic suggestions can be used to reinforce this point and enables the client to recognize foods that help to make them feel good inside. As the client becomes more and more in tune with their own body, they move towards gaining a strong sense of inner security and confidence.

Many people gain weight due to a series of bad habits they develop over the years. This may include reaching for biscuits with a cup of tea, driving short distances instead of walking or eating heavy meals late at night. Clients will find it easier to change habits when they become consciously aware that they are not a part of themselves, but simply bits of behaviour that they have learnt and can be unlearnt. Hypnotherapeutic suggestions can help clients break old habits on an unconscious level. Suggestions can be made during the hypnotherapy session to incorporate new patterns of behaviour with regard to times, places and reasons for eating. Post-hypnotic suggestions can be incorporated into the hypnotherapy session for: symptom substitution, trading one eating habit for another healthier option; symptom amelioration, to directly reduce overeating and symptom utilization, to encourage the client to accept and re-define eating habits (Alman 1992).

There are some people for whom being overweight is a symptom of something deeper and the therapist may use analytical tools such as regression or dissociation. However, the vast majority of people who seek hypnotherapy for weight control, respond very well to suggestion therapy combined with goal-setting visualizations and techniques to listen and respond to their own specific and unique body. This combination can help the client to gain control over their eating patterns and develop a more positive body image.

BODY IMAGE AND SEXUAL ISSUES RELATING TO ILLNESS OR DISABILITY

Changes arising due to illness or disability can leave patients and their partners requiring support to adjust to the body image and sexual issues which may arise. Any support offered should aim to facilitate adjustment

Body image, sexuality, weight loss and hypnotherapy

to the resulting changes and the losses which these may bring. Each patient's response to his or her illness is unique, and helping them through the anxiety of adjustment requires an individualized holistic approach. People use different coping mechanisms in an effort to adjust and an initial reaction of denial has an important role in protecting against unbearable anxiety (Wells 2000). Before using any hypnotherapy techniques, the therapist needs to assess if this is the case and decide whether hypnotherapy at this time would have a positive effect. In many cases, denial operates as a healthy mechanism and protects the person against the immediate shock of reality (Cawthorn 2006). Davidhizar and Giger (1998: 44) remind us that 'normally denial diminishes and the person begins to face and accept the harsh reality of what has been blocked'. However, when denial appears to be causing a problem or is longstanding, often the solution lies in identifying and working through what is causing the blockage. The patient's own critical sensor will protect them if they are not ready to make any changes during trance work.

CANCER DIAGNOSIS

Being diagnosed with cancer can have a major impact on body image and can include a total body effect, as patients come to terms with their own mortality (see Ch. 14). The psychological impact of an altered appearance relating to cancer can be far-reaching and varied (Harcourt & Ramsey 2006). This is because problems occur not only in relation to the disease, but also as a result of the side-effects of treatments, which include surgery, chemotherapy and radiotherapy and hormone therapy. For these reasons, people may be attempting to recover from one body image change, only to be faced with one after another, which makes adjustment even more difficult.

When adjusting to body image changes, the reactions of others are very important. This is particularly relevant if the changes arise as a result of rapid disease, surgery, accidents and cancer treatments, as the person is still struggling to come to terms with their own thoughts and feelings surrounding this. John Diamond (1998) wrote extensively about the ongoing problems he experienced in relation to his oral cancer and subsequent surgery, chemotherapy and radiotherapy. He reminds us that the negative reactions of others can inadvertently add to the problems.

Diamond (1998) writes about his responses to individual treatments. He recalls his surprise at his reaction to the loss of body hair during chemotherapy and the psychological effect this had on his manhood. He goes on to say how he was unprepared for the anger which erupted from nowhere when receiving radiotherapy and the sadness and regret that this was often directed at the ones closest to him, who were his wife and children.

Body image problems (including sexual problems) can occur in relation to any form of cancer, affecting both males and females. Many women report feeling less sexually attractive following breast surgery, as breasts are often seen as a symbol of femininity and sexual attractiveness (Burwell et al 2006). Chemotherapy can add to the problem due to hair loss and increased weight. Breast Cancer Care (2008) sums up the difficulties experienced by this client group in a quote by a patient who was undergoing chemotherapy, who when asked about her sexuality said:

She didn't feel too sexually attractive as a sweating, bald-headed one breasted woman with mouth ulcers and sore gums!

Men also have body image and sexual problems relating to effects of surgery and hormone therapy for prostate cancer. Reduced fertility, and altered sexual identity or masculinity being just a few of the problems which can arise. There are many issues relating to this client group, which are covered in more detail by White et al (2006).

For some people, the whole experience of any disabling illness can have a profound effect on their sense of self. They effectively become defined by the disease which can potentially take on a life of its own. These thoughts may be out of their conscious awareness, which can lead on to very limiting beliefs about themselves, and translate into changes in behaviour. One common behaviour is avoidance. It is useful to use hypnotherapy techniques when working with patients, as often in trance they elicit a strong image of the disease. It is useful to gain their permission to elicit the image and what this feels like. Some people describe its shape, colour and texture very easily before a trance state is induced, while others only become aware of what it looks like during trance. Negotiation is the key to working in this way, as the person may not want to change the image or bring it into their current awareness through the use of hypnotherapy.

An example of how this approach was effective is with a young woman who learned to adjust and accommodate a tumour situated too near her spine to safely remove it (see Case study 2, Box 9.3).

SELF-ESTEEM AND SELF-WORTH

Low self-esteem and/or self-worth can result from body image problems. However, these could be longstanding issues which the new problems further compound. Newell (1999) suggests that body image changes can affect the person's quality of life, resulting in reduced self-confidence and low self-esteem, which in turn can cause difficult social interactions and, ultimately, social withdrawal. White (2006: 678) reminds us that 'serious illness and disability remove a person from their accustomed personal, social and sexual relation, threatening self-esteem and attractiveness at a time when their need for intimacy and belonging may be greatest'.

When assessing patients, it is important to elicit their perception of the problem and also find out how significant others perceive it. Perceptions are important and patients often assume that their body image changes will be problematic for their partner, when in reality this is not usually the case. A Macmillan 'super survey' (2008) found that only 5% of partners found the patient's body image change to be problematic (see: www.macmillan.org. uk/sex).

It is important to assess the patient's mood, as a low mood can impact on their body image, self-esteem and self-worth. Common psychological problems include anxiety, depression and adjustment problems/disorders. People living with depression often have negative expectancy and Yapko (2001) suggests that the first task in treating a depressed client is to address any sense of hopelessness.

BOX 9.3 Case study 2

Kirsty, aged 24, came for hypnotherapy to help her to adjust psychologically and physically to a tumour within her abdomen. During imagery she saw the tumour as black and impacting on her femininity (see Fig. 9.1). She sat awkwardly and because of this complained of low back pain. In trance she was able to clear the black away and pack the area around the tumour with white feathers, making it much softer and accommodating. This resulted in her being able to sit in a more relaxed way, reducing her back pain. Hypnotherapy was used to work on an abusive relationship, and she was happy to send the abuser off in a hot air balloon. Kirsty went on to draw this work in collaboration with her art therapist. The internal changes can be seen in Figures 9.1 and 9.2 and her personal growth and healing can be seen in Figures 9.3 and 9.4. She still has the tumour *in situ* (currently dormant) but has adjusted to the disability it brings.

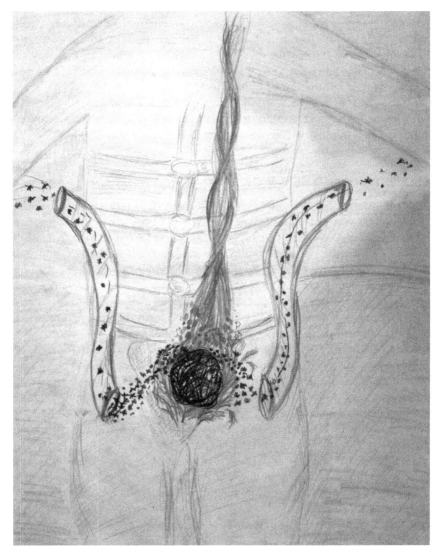

FIG 9.1 Imagery. Kirsty, Case study 2 (see Box 9.3 for details).

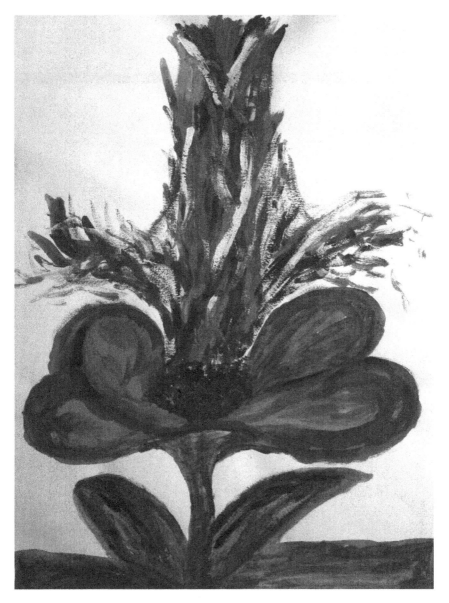

FIG 9.2 Imagery. Kirsty, Case study 2 (see Box 9.3 for details).

SECURITY

Personal security is something we do not consider when life is going well and it is only when our security is challenged by life-threatening or life-changing experiences that we become aware of it. At these times, our whole being is threatened and we begin to consider our own mortality. An example where both individual and collective security was threatened was following the 9/11 or 7/7 terrorist attacks. During this time, there was a sense of personal and collective insecurity, which took time for people to adjust and

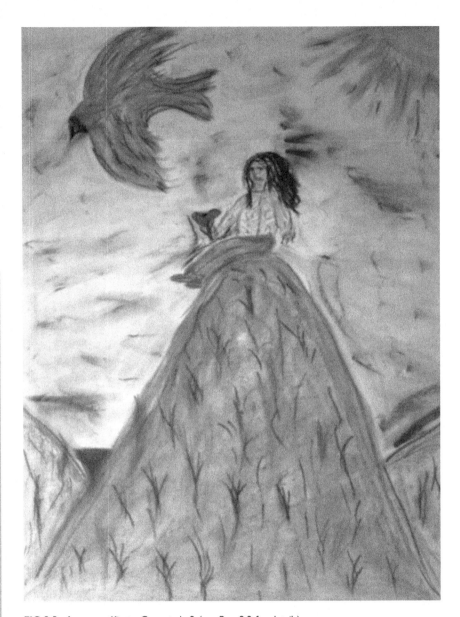

FIG 9.3 Imagery. Kirsty, Case study 2 (see Box 9.3 for details).

move on from. This same scenario is repeated following the diagnosis of a life-threatening or life-limiting illness and can impact on the personal security of both the patient and their family members. From an existential perspective, cancer is still (incorrectly) viewed by many to signify impending death. John Diamond (1998) wrote that when diagnosed with cancer, he saw a death sentence. For him this eventually became true, but for many, it merely raises existential concerns which need to be worked through (see Ch. 14). Illness may bring other issues which relate to security such as

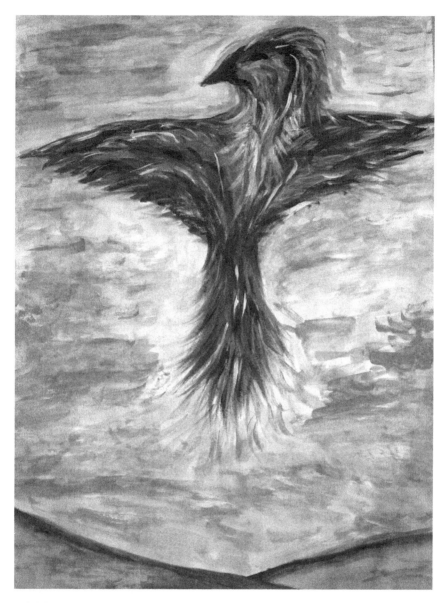

FIG 9.4 Imagery. Kirsty, Case study 2 (see Box 9.3 for details).

financial, social, role changes and the ability to maintain and develop relationships. It may also raise old insecurities which can be transformed through trance (see Case study 3, Box 9.4).

Maintaining security is important for a healthy body image, and hypnotherapy techniques which help patients regain their sense of security and regain control are of great benefit. Learning self-hypnosis, accessing a safe place and having a supply of positive good memories which can be anchored at times of insecurity can all be useful. Being able to change an insecure image can also help to increase security.

> **BOX 9.4 Case study 3**
>
> Sheila, a 50-year-old lady, was recovering from breast surgery and she was afraid to undress in front of her husband in case he said she was 'ugly'. On inquiry, it transpired that her mother had called her ugly as a teenager and this is where her body image issues originated. In order to reduce the impact of this memory, an adapted NLP technique was used (Rushworth 1999). Sheila contained the image of her mother (saying she was ugly) in a television screen. Sheila had the control switch and she turned the colour down, making it black and white, then turned the sound down and finally shrunk the picture down until she was happy with it. At the following session, Sheila said that her mother (surprisingly) had made contact with her for the first time in 20 years. Sheila was able to meet her and saw that her unkind words no longer impacted on her. When Sheila realized she was projecting her mother's behaviour on to her husband, she allowed him to see her naked without fear of rejection.

LOSS

It is important to identify and work with the losses which a change in body image may bring. These losses could be overt and may include loss of body part/s following surgery including amputation, mastectomy, or enucleation of an eye. Other less overt losses, but equally significant, may include hysterectomy, oophorectomy (ovaries), prostatectomy and total or hemi-colectomy. Losses which relate to bodily functions such as colostomy, ileostomy and urostomy, cause the loss of the person's ability to function as a normal human being. All losses need to be grieved for and many people are able to do this for themselves, while others need psychological support in order to achieve this. However, some people will need additional support in the form of hypnotherapy in order to adjust to the changes which the loss has brought about.

SEXUAL ABUSE/TRAUMA

When assessing people with body image or sexual concerns, it is important to consider that some may have a history of sexual abuse or trauma. These patients may present with body image issues, low mood or anxiety disorders, low self-worth or poor self-esteem, or be treated for an illness which is directly or indirectly linked to the abuse. Personal clinical practice has involved working with people who have developed cervical, vulval, ovarian, uterine or anal cancer, some of which may be linked to earlier sexual experiences or abuse. Some patients do not overtly make the link, but for those who do, this can add to the distress they are already experiencing. Fortunately, there are hypnotherapy techniques which can prove useful with this client group if they are comfortable working in this way.

When working with patients it is important to listen to how they tell the narrative relating to their concerns. The 'clean language' approach adopted by Grove and Panzer (1991) allows the meaning attached to the abuse/trauma to be the patient's and not the therapist's. If denial is evident and it is proving to be a useful coping mechanism, then this should be respected.

However, if the memories are problematic, there are a number of techniques which can transform them into more positive ones where the patient regains control. Grove and Panzer (1991) suggest a variety of ways when working in this area, all of which should match up with the person's memories, language, symbols and metaphors.

Negative images can be changed using hypnotherapy techniques. Patients can help to repair the damage by using imagery to heal the areas which they feel have been damaged. They can be supported to imagine themselves regaining control in a situation where this was not the case. If they want to change the image of a perpetrator, they can make them look silly, or shrink them down in size, or send them off in a hot air balloon. This can be achieved during trance (see Case studies 2 and 3, Boxes 9.3 and 9.4).

Where patients have unpleasant memories which they do not want to re-live, then an NLP technique adapted from Rushworth (1999) can safely wipe the memory without the patient needing to re-visit it or talk it through with the therapist. The technique currently used in practice is as follows:

1. The therapist talks through the process with the patient before inducing trance.
2. The patient will be invited to find a safe place, and in this place they will go into a cinema where they can play a film (backwards) of the traumatic event.
3. Before they do this they will have anchored good memories in which they felt safe and secure; one from before the trauma and one from after the trauma.
4. They will be invited to run a film/video of the traumatic event, backwards and forwards until it is wiped. In order to run the film they will be invited to float out of their body, so they will be watching themselves watching the film (disassociation).
5. If during this process they need any support, they will be able to use the adult part of their personality to comfort the distressed part.

Patients will only consent to this technique if they are comfortable with how it is set up with the therapist. It can have a very healing effect without the therapist needing to talk through (or indeed know) what the trauma entailed. They are merely a companion while the patient transforms their negative image.

Working with dreams

Another way of working with trauma is to work with the dreams or nightmares which patients recall. Mallon (2001, 2003) and Kearney and Richardson (2006) offer suggestions as to how to work with dreams, and these have been integrated into the authors' clinical practice. They recommend avoiding over-interpretation, allowing the person to make their own sense of what the dream evokes and the symbols and feelings they contain. If the patient is comfortable recalling their dream, this can be undertaken within the therapy session or through keeping a dream diary. This involves drawing or giving a narrative of the dreams, noting the shapes, colours, whether any patterns emerge and whether the dreams are reoccurring.

Mallon (2001) suggests that a number of questions are asked in relation to the dream. These refer to who was in the dream and where was it set. If the patient was in it, were they active or passive? Was there anything which impressed them or disturbed them about the dream and what was the main feeling? Healing can sometimes come in sharing the dream. However, for many patients, if there are negative images, traumatic scenes or incomplete or difficult endings, then to transform these while in trance can be very healing. If the dream relates to an actual situation, then it is useful to inquire what the patient wants to change within the dream; whether this is images, symbols or feelings, or even having permission to say to another person what they feel is important for them to hear. If this is carefully set up, then the patient, while in trance, is usually able to achieve a positive outcome with the therapist as their companion. In practice, patients usually know how they would like the ending to be.

Many dreams do not relate to any particular event. However, they may be a metaphor for something else and in recalling the dream, the link may become clearer. One dream which patients commonly recall is one where they are in toilets, where there is no privacy, where cubicle doors are missing and when they report this to people who should be able to help, they are not believed. Sometimes this symbolizes how they feel about their treatment, that what should be personal and hidden is revealed to anyone and everyone, with little regard for how that impacts on their privacy. In addition, despite telling people who should have been able to help, they were not believed, which mirrored their actual experience.

CONCLUSION

In conclusion, having looked at body image and the role it has in health as well as illness, this appears to be an important aspect in society, health and social care. The current obsession with the perfect body is difficult for most people to achieve. Added to this, the negative body image changes brought on by ageing, accidents or illness, can further reduce a patient's self-esteem and self-worth. Weight gain is an additional problem in relation to body image and this has also been addressed, along with sexual abuse and trauma. A number of assessment models and hypnotherapeutic approaches have been explored and these have been linked to personal case studies.

REFERENCES

Alman, B., 1992. Self-hypnosis. The complete guide to better health and self-change. Souvenir Press, London.

American Society for Clinical Hypnosis, 2009. Information for the general public. Online. Available: http://asch.net/genpublicinfo.htm.

Barraclough, J., 1999. Cancer and emotion, a practical guide to psycho-oncology, third ed. John Wiley, Chichester.

Berne, E., 1972. What do you say after you say hello? Bantam Books, New York.

Breast Cancer Care, 2008. Sexuality, intimacy and breast cancer. BCC, London.

Burwell, S.R., Case, L.D., Kaelin, C., et al., 2006. Sexual problems in younger women after breast cancer surgery. J. Clin. Oncol. 24 (18), 2815–2821.

Cash, T.F., Pruzinsky, T. (Eds.), 2002. Body image: a handbook of theory, research and clinical practice. Guildford Press, New York.

Cawthorn, A., 2006. Working with the denied body. In: Mackereth, P., Carter, A. (Eds.), Massage & bodywork: adapting therapies for cancer care. Churchill Livingstone, Edinburgh.

Cunningham, A.J., 2000. The healing journey: overcoming the crisis of cancer. Key Porter Books, Toronto.

Davidhizar, R., Giger, J.N., 1998. Patient's use of denial: coping with the unacceptable. Nurs. Stand. 12 (43), 44–46.

Diamond, J., 1998. C: because cowards get cancer too. Phoenix Books, London.

Freud, S., 1936. Sexuality and the psychology of love. Simon & Schuster, New York.

Grogan, S., 1999. Body image. Routledge, London.

Grove, D.J., Panzer, B.I., 1991. Resolving traumatic memories. Metaphors and symbols in psychotherapy. Irvington, New York.

Harcourt, D., Ramsey, N., 2006. Altered body image. In: Kearney, N., Richardson, A. (Eds.), Nursing patients with cancer principles and practice. Elsevier, Edinburgh.

Mallon, B., 2001. Venus dreaming. A guide to women's dreams and nightmares. Newleaf, Dublin.

Mallon, B., 2003. The dream bible. Godsfield Press, Hampshire.

Newell, R.J., 1999. Altered body image: a fear-avoidance model of psycho-social difficulties following disfigurement. J. Adv. Nurs. 30, 1230–1238.

NICE, 2004. Supportive and palliative care guidelines. National Institute for Clinical Excellence, London. Online. Available: www.nice.org.uk.

Orbach, S., 2009. Bodies. Profile Books, London.

Price, B., 1990. Body image. Nursing concepts and care. Prentice Hall, New Jersey.

Rushworth, C., 1999. Making a difference in cancer care: practical techniques in palliative and curative treatment, second ed. Souvenir Press, London.

Stephenson, K., 2005. Slimmer fitter healthier audio CD booklet. Innerchange Programmes.

Webster's New World Medical Dictionary, third ed. 2008. Wiley, Hoboken, NJ.

Wells, D. (Ed.), 2000. Caring for sexuality in health care. Churchill Livingstone, Edinburgh.

White, I., 2006. The impact of cancer and cancer therapy on sexual and reproductive health. In: Kearney, N., Richardson, A. (Eds.), Nursing patients with cancer: principles and practice. Elsevier, Edinburgh.

Yapko, 2001. Treating depression with hypnosis integrating cognitive – behavioural and strategic approaches. Routledge, Philadelphia.

USEFUL RESOURCES

Changing Faces, 1–2 Junction Mews, London, W2 IPN, UK – a charity which helps people trying to cope with disfigurement. Tel: 020 7706 4232; e-mail: info@changingfaces.co.uk, website: www.changing faces.co.uk.

Let's Face It, 14 Fallowfield, Yately, Hampshire GU46 6LW, UK – offers a support network for anyone affected by facial disfigurement.

Menopausal Matters—Helpline 0845 122 8616; e-mail: daisy@daisynetwork.org.uk.
www.macmillan.org.uk/sex.
www.learnzone.macmillan.org.uk.
www.cancerbackup.org.uk/
Resourcessupport/
Relationshipscommunication/Sexuality.

Body image, sexuality, weight loss and hypnotherapy

10 Helping a person go *Smoke Free*: a reflective approach

Lynne Tomlinson • Paula Maycock • Peter A. Mackereth

CHAPTER OUTLINE

This chapter was constructed to firmly place those jaded smoking cessation scripts where they belong. Becoming 'smoke free' can be a challenging and creative process which, like a duet, requires therapist and client to work in harmony. A SEEDING model for use with complementary therapy interventions is presented and explored. Case studies are included to illustrate how clients can be facilitated and supported. Reflective practice exercises are offered to assist you to review and integrate what you have learnt both consciously and subconsciously. We hope that once you have read this chapter you will lapse into reverie and consider your role in smoking cessation in a new and exciting way. Absorb, learn and utilize the following information at a pace that is entirely appropriate for you, so that you can become more confident about your fluency and potency as a therapist.

© 2010 Elsevier Ltd.
DOI: 10.1016/B978-0-7020-3082-6.00012-5

KEY WORDS

Smoking cessation
Cravings
SEEDING model
Reflective practice
Self-efficacy

INTRODUCTION

Integrative hypnotherapy incorporates complementary therapies to create an individualized and client-led approach to smoking cessation. Hypnotherapy alone has been reported to assist people to feel engaged and empowered in the process of smoking cessation (Ahijevych 2000). A review of the non-pharmacological research literature suggests that smoking cessation can be helped through a structured programme of support from health professionals (Lancaster et al 2000), which can also be assisted by the use of auricular acupuncture (White et al 2000) (Fig. 10.1A). Massage and reflexology (Fig. 10.1B) have also been claimed to support patients in managing cravings in combination with standard nicotine replacement therapies (Hernandez-Reif et al 1999, Maycock & Mackereth 2009). In a clinical environment, this heady mix of interventions may confound some practitioners used to a mono-therapy approach. Inevitably, critics demand evidence for each element of such a complex package and integrative hypnotherapy provides scope for quality research endeavours. World tobacco control initiatives include protecting people from passive smoking, offering support to people who want to stop smoking and warning and informing people about the dangers of tobacco (Bala et al 2008). The challenge is how these objectives can be achieved in a therapy room. It is hoped that the reflective practices (which help unfold each element of the SEEDING model) and the real case studies that demonstrate an integrative approach will help therapists cultivate qualities, such as flexibility, empathy and curiosity, in order to help them assist their clients to become 'smoke free'.

THE SEEDING MODEL

Jay Haley first introduced the concept of 'seeding' in *Uncommon Therapy* (1973), based on his analysis of the work of Milton H. Erickson. Haley noted that Erickson would seed or establish ideas and refer back to them several times during a session or series of sessions to create a specific response-set (conditioned behavioural responses) that could evoke a powerful and appropriate response to a given suggestion. Seeding is not unique to hypnotherapy, it is also known as 'priming' when employed by social psychologists or 'foreshadowing' when used as a plot device in literature or films (Zeig 1990).

The SEEDING model, as illustrated below, is more than a handy acronym to remember effective and powerful elements of integrative hypnotherapy. Seeding can take place at many levels during a hypnotherapy session and

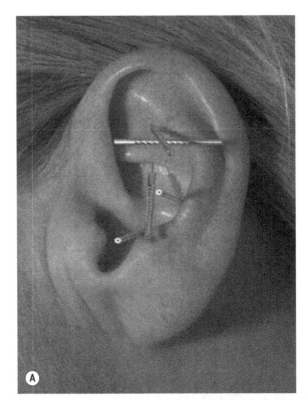

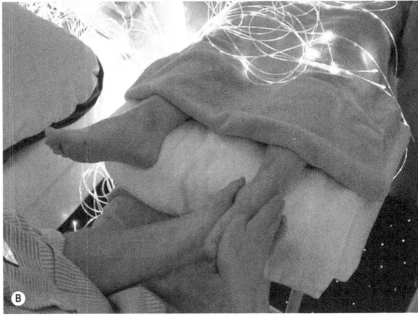

FIG 10.1 Supportive interventions for smoking cessation. (A) Auricular acupuncture and (B) reflexology.

> **BOX 10.1 SEEDING Model for integrated hypnotherapy practice**
>
> 1. Selecting: appropriate information and interventions
> 2. Empathizing: understanding feelings, motives and situations
> 3. Empowering: client choice and client actions
> 4. Diffusing: anxiety, stress and cravings
> 5. Installing: new behaviours, resources and feelings
> 6. Negotiating: conscious and subconscious objections to change
> 7. Gathering: momentum and desire for a smoke-free future.

can also be used as a pre-hypnotic technique that requires strategy or a therapeutic 'planning ahead' and starts from the moment of contact with your client. Geary (1994) suggests that seeding can also occur on multiple levels with pauses, tonality, volume, inflection, gestures, word-play and even postural changes. The macro and micro applications are limited only by the ability and imagination of the therapist.

The SEEDING model presented in Box 10.1 creates a menu of therapeutic interventions that can be used selectively (as each can evoke or 'seed' a useful response-set) or in a synergistic combination where each seed will reinforce the other. There will inevitably be some overlap between elements but this also provides opportunities for consolidation and review. You may feel that some of the reflective practice exercises could be more appropriately used within a different element of the model. Feel free to customize and use as creatively as you wish. At the end of this chapter, you may like to think how to 'grow' the model for your own practice.

REFLECTIVE PRACTICE

Reflective practice, as defined by Schön (1983), involves carefully considering real world experiences and linking knowledge to practice. This is a continuous process of reviewing professional practice, which can be facilitated, supported or coached through supervisory, mentoring or preceptorship arrangements (Morton-Cooper & Palmer 2000). Models of reflective practice have been developed to guide practitioners in the process. These can include frameworks and/or cyclical processes (Gibbs 1988, Johns 2004), which ask questions, such as: 'What happened?', 'How might you respond differently next time?', 'What are the ethical and/or professional issues raised by the situation?'. The goal of any model is not to be prescriptive, rather to enable the professional to grow their practice. Using the SEEDING model we have devised a series of questions (these are not exhaustive) for therapists to use 'in' and 'reflect on' smoking cessation practice. The model, case study examples and reflective practice points are summarized in Table 10.1.

This model is not an attempt to itemize reflective practice, force interventions into arbitrary stages or be rigidly adhered to. You may feel that some of the reflective practice exercises could be more appropriately used within a different element of the model – feel free to customize and use as creatively as you wish. As Johns (2002: 17) suggests, a model can help the therapist to bring together 'fragments of experience into a meaningful whole'.

Table 10.1 *The SEEDING model, reflective practices and illustrative case studies*

Element of model	Area of focus	Reflective aim	Case study
Selecting	Consider yourself Consider the client	To find the appropriate information and interventions for the session	Rozia
Empathizing	Understanding feelings Images and reactions Sensation and intensity The therapeutic process	Learning to understand feelings, motives and situations	Mark
Empowering	Clients, yourself and colleagues	To enhance client choice and the actions they choose to take and to consider your working environment	James
Diffusing	The client as the 'expert' Finding exceptions Finding what works	To understand the anxieties or difficulties that behavioural change can evoke	Robert
Installing	'Imagine if …' Finding something compulsive 'Seek and you will find'	To find new behaviours, resources and feelings that will help the client to achieve his/her therapy aim	Alison
Negotiating	Smoking 'but(s)' Clearing the way for change Something came up	To identify objections to change at all levels and find a more skilful way of responding to them	Hannah
Gathering	'Ready, steady, go …' Bespoke suggestions Time for a change	Generating energy, momentum and desire to change	Dave

1. SELECTING: APPROPRIATE INFORMATION AND INTERVENTIONS

As an integrative therapist working in a variety of settings, it can be a challenge to negotiate between the individual needs of the client and the environment in which smoking cessation is offered. Most smokers know that smoking is harmful, expensive and unpleasant. They may also feel jaded by the repetition of questions that they may have been asked before and the offer of leaflets, brochures and 'advice' that often repeats what they already know. For therapists, there might be a requirement to record specific data about a client's smoking behaviour or complete a checklist of information/interventions provided, regardless of client needs, in order to fulfil important clinical or funding requirements. In addition, certain safety protocols may need to be observed before hypnotherapy, acupuncture, aromatherapy, reflexology and other complementary therapies can be used. Information gathering in the process of completing essential documentation can be a wonderful opportunity to come alongside the person, create rapport and a space to seed options for change.

In reality, smoking cessation leaflets may be unwelcomed or not given at the right time, with the result that they are put aside without being read. This is despite local and national printed smoking cessation materials being highly accessible, multi-lingual and quality controlled, with useful contact details and advice on the safe use of pharmacological and non-pharmacological products. They can also act as an aide memoire or positive reinforcement to the client's desire to stop smoking. For smokers who have high health literacy, or would prefer to work privately and in their own way, this could be the information and intervention of choice. A good knowledge of the contents of any smoking cessation material provided can help the therapist to 'tailor' information or refer to specific parts that could interest or motivate. This tailoring sends a powerful message to the client that their needs are being listened to carefully. For those smokers taking the first tentative steps towards becoming smoke-free and 'checking out' the service, the offer of a booklet with a warm smile (even on the telephone you can tell when someone smiles) can anchor (a stimulus linked to a specific feeling or behavioural response) positive associations. It is important, professionally, for all therapists working in smoking cessation to have an understanding of conventional approaches, and be aware of developments in pharmacological treatments. National smoking cessation reports and guidelines are available, with research reviews and recommendations for smoking cessation practice, available online (see Further Reading and Resources).

Reflective practice 1

This practice is designed to engage the therapist in a process of identifying what information/help might be needed to make a change in an individual's health behaviours. The therapist is then invited to consider how a client might undertake a similar process (see Boxes 10.2 and 10.3).

BOX 10.2

Consider yourself
- Take some time to think about a health change you would like to make that feels important to you. Identify what information is needed for you to consider making those changes. In selecting the most helpful approach, what would you discard immediately and what would you hold onto?

Consider the client
- How do you know when your clients are ready to hear and seek information? How could you make smoking cessation information relevant, compelling and fresh? How could that information be 'seeded' by pre-hypnotic suggestions?

BOX 10.3 Case study 1

Rozia, aged 49 years, attended an acupuncture clinic for support in dealing with hot flushes, and started a conversation with her therapist regarding smoking. She stated that she had no desire to stop but was happy to accept a leaflet about the services offered by the clinic. The therapist warmly honoured her choice and stopped all discussion about smoking other than to ask permission to write their name and direct contact number on the leaflet. Rozia, 12 months later, returned to the clinic and specifically requested the therapist by name to discuss nicotine replacement therapy (NRT) and acupuncture for smoking cessation.

2. EMPATHIZING: UNDERSTANDING FEELINGS, MOTIVES AND SITUATIONS

National stop smoking campaigns ensure that smoking remains highly visible as a political, social and ecological issue. They also promote social change by affecting social norms and values about smoking (Wellings et al 2000). For many smokers, the issue of 'social smoking' can be more to do with shame, isolation and conflict. How smokers perceive themselves can result in 'negative affect' (negative emotions such as anxiety, guilt and depression) and a lack of 'self-efficacy', resulting in feeling unable to achieve goals. This requires a skilful and delicate touch from the therapist, as these issues, if not addressed, can undermine the therapy process and your client's perceived ability to achieve a smoke-free lifestyle. Consider for example the much used phrase 'willpower'. This nebulous and unhelpful term and the supposed 'lack of willpower' is often used in judgement by others against smokers during their stopping process and can even become part of a client's own negative self-talk. It is also disempowering. Human beings stop smoking, not the 'willpower'.

Reflective practice 2

This practice is designed to sensitize you (as therapist) to some of the social issues facing smokers. It will also help you and your clients to explore the construction of internal dialogues, images and sensations (see Boxes 10.4 and 10.5).

BOX 10.4

Understanding feelings
▪ Where do you think your beliefs about smoking have come from? Do you feel part of a majority or part of a minority? Does that support or undermine you?

Images and reactions
▪ Imagine smokers in different situations. For example: a child, pregnant woman or patient on a drip, smoking (you may think of others). Notice your reaction and any judgements aroused.

Sensation and intensity
▪ Notice the key perceptual modalities and sub-modalities that affect your experience. Play with the 'master controls' such as brightness, distance, volume, clarity, sensation, taste, smell, etc. Write down the 'controls' that work best for you.

In the therapeutic process ...
▪ Ask and note how your client describes/constructs/uses modalities to report his/her feelings about smoking. Observe any incongruence between your client's tone and his/her non-verbal behaviours. It may be helpful to develop an 'ear' that is mindful of disparaging language, dismissive gestures, negative tones and other behaviours that reveal negative self-concepts. How could you use these observations and insights within the therapy process?

> **BOX 10.5 Case study 2**
>
> Mark, aged 52 with stomach cancer and attached to an intravenous infusion, was approached by a member of staff while smoking outside the hospital door. He was being told about the smoking cessation service when a passing visitor interrupted their conversation saying 'about time . . . this is a hospital'. A few days later he came to the smoking cessation clinic. On talking about his motivation to attend, he snapped 'some bloke got at me while I was outside having a cig'. Mark's therapist replied 'you have obviously given it some thought and decided to take action'. We can help you manage your smoking while you're in hospital . . . you decide when to stop . . . we can also offer you support to reduce stress.
>
> Mark chose to use the NRT inhaler to manage cravings and HypnoReflexology© for stress reduction and well-being. During the treatment, Mark revealed that the stranger's comment had made him feel 'ashamed to the point of tears'. The therapist supported Mark by using gentle ego strengthening suggestions to promote feelings of self-efficacy, to help him acknowledge his ability to make changes and neutralize the feelings of shame.

3. EMPOWERING: CLIENT CHOICE AND CLIENT ACTIONS

True empowerment means that clients have the power, information, resources and abilities to make their own choices about what they want to do. This element of the seeding model is also at the heart of integrative hypnotherapy and requires a high level of self-knowledge, authenticity and trust. As therapists, we may work within a clinical environment with its own agenda or hold strong beliefs or opinions (or work in association with other therapists that do) about our 'success rates', that smoking is an addiction or just a habit; the use of NRT and pharmacotherapies; cutting down and stopping; or even the allocation of NHS resources to patients who have a smoking-related illness. These can all affect how we respond to the client's choice about how or when they choose to stop smoking. We also work with conscious and subconscious awareness and need to remain especially mindful of how we ethically manipulate verbal and non-verbal suggestions. Consider the selection of certain words, the subtle stresses and tonality, pace and pauses and how powerful these qualities are. For therapists using touch therapies and/or acupuncture, as well as hypnotherapy, the sheer quantity of simultaneous communication channels can mean that any incongruence between the words and intent of the therapist (or therapists working in conflict) could easily be 'felt' by the client.

Reflective practice 3

This practice is designed to elicit self-awareness. There are no correct or incorrect answers. However, it may intrigue you to see how your beliefs can change or intensify and how this in turn informs your working practice. We invite you to repeat this reflective exercise as often as you wish. It helps to keep a diary or take these reflections to your supervision sessions (see Boxes 10.6 and 10.7).

BOX 10.6

Clients: their values, beliefs and attitudes

- How would you feel about working with a client who only wants to reduce his/her intake, use NRT to 'get them through a day or two', or stop smoking temporarily?
- Are there any clients you would prefer to work with . . . or not work with?

Yourself and colleagues

- Are you more comfortable (and successful) if your client's beliefs and views on smoking are in accord with your own (e.g. addiction or habit debate). Do you sense a desire to want to correct their misunderstanding/views?
- How do you respond to colleagues and other therapists who hold different views from you about the 'best' interventions and support for smoking cessation?
- What evidence do you have to support your own working practices? How did your training influence your working practice? What are your attitudes to NRT and pharmacotherapies?
- How would you deal with a referral made by someone other than the patient requesting smoking cessation?

BOX 10.7 Case study 3

A surgeon requested smoking cessation services for James, a preoperative patient, but had not received his consent to do so. He was thanked for his concern and thoroughness in providing support for James but was informed that it was policy to contact only those patients who had specifically given consent. He relayed this to James who rang our services directly and confirmed his desire to stop smoking but only once he was in the hospital. James did not wish to stop before the operation but was happy to receive support, advice and be taught self-hypnosis to help prepare him. James stopped smoking while in hospital and remained smoke free at a 12 week follow-up call.

4. DIFFUSING: ANXIETY, STRESS AND CRAVINGS

In 2006, 68% of smokers said that they would like to stop smoking with 59% stating that it would be very or fairly difficult to stop for a whole day (General Household Survey 2006). Human beings tend to smoke for specific reasons and most smokers have a cigarette suitable for all occasions! Many therapists feel that, as part of their educative role, they need to point out the inconsistencies between what smoking and nicotine are doing to the body and what physical or emotional effect the client is reporting. In essence, this is 'correcting' the client's perception but which reality will remain the most powerful or compelling? A broader perspective invites the question: 'Is there a need to be right and how, specifically, is this part of integrative hypnotherapy?'. Rather than locking into a dialogue that could result in opposition, it can be more useful to consider the context or situation where a person feels they need to smoke and identify exceptions to their 'normal' smoking behaviour. The therapeutic alliance can then be built by collaborating on the common ground of these exceptions. Each exception can be utilized as a resource without antagonism or contradiction and the smoker remains the 'expert' on their own smoking behaviour.

Although anxiety, stress and strong emotions feature in the narrative of many smokers, there are also smokers who share 'peak' moments such as intense pleasure, achievement or post-orgasm with their cigarette. How therapists co-create, with their clients, a substitute that is as flexible as their cigarettes are perceived to be is part of the beauty and challenge of the work.

Integrative hypnotherapy provides many opportunities to work with the 'body' and 'spirit' as well as the mind. Holding, nurturing, supporting and connecting with clients on all these levels is possible. These gentle and human qualities can enhance and work synergistically with solution-focused or cognitive approaches to hypnotherapy. These supportive and complementary therapies can include massage, reflexology, aromatherapy and acupunctures. There is good evidence for the efficacy of interventions on well-being, anxiety and mood (see Chs 7 and 8).

Many hypnotherapists dismiss cravings as short-lived phenomena that are a result of nicotine withdrawal and concentrate on removing all cravings with direct suggestion. Standardized scripts for smoking cessation place considerable emphasis on 'denying cravings'. Such approaches can build in therapeutic limitations or even failure if they do not match client reality and do not allow for dynamic development. Time spent identifying client resources, matching to situations, cognitive-behavioural interventions, teaching relaxation techniques and creating powerful anchors will help to set the client up for success in the short term and allow for the inevitable changes on his/her smoke-free journey. Finding and testing more flexible behaviours than smoking provides a systematic way to deal with objections to stopping smoking at all levels of awareness. Some of the techniques taught may naturally lead into altered states and so can be tested both consciously and while in trance. The identification and testing of such strategies takes time and energy, so therapists need to consider whether long, short, single session or multi-session approaches to smoking cessation are needed, rather than a 'one-size-fits-all' contract.

Reflective practice 4

This section is designed to help you put reflection into practice and more importantly, to maintain an on-going reflective quality while you are working to identify client resources, strengthen rapport and design/test interventions. This ongoing process can enhance your sense of congruence, authenticity and connect you to your intuitive 'knowing'. It is also an acknowledgement of your potency as a therapist. Just as in all trance work, pauses and silences in dialogue can create nurturing and respectful spaces for both therapist and client to just take time to journey within and find responses, at all levels of awareness. Aromas add a sensory quality to the therapeutic work. They can linger, resonate and harmonize with the suggestions offered – whether vocally, or with touch. You just have to think of the taste of a lemon, the colours of a lavender field and the smell of roses (see Boxes 10.8 and 10.9).

BOX 10.8

The client as the expert

- Ask your clients to teach you how to smoke just like them. How do they know when it's time for a cigarette? What do they notice in their body? What images do they make in their mind's eye? Do they talk to themselves? What do they become aware of in their environment? How do they interact with others? Explore and record all of their modalities of experience. Are there any differences between a cigarette for pleasure and a cigarette for unpleasant emotions? What are the similarities?

Finding exceptions to the rules

- Apart from a cigarette, what does your client identify that would be helpful in trigger situations. Have they ever got through a situation similar to the 'trigger' occasion without a cigarette? How did they do it? How would they like to do it?

Finding what works

- In hypnosis, repeat back exception behaviour scenarios and use ideomotor responses (IMRs) to obtain feedback on their efficacy. Anchor resource states and test both in trance and on emergence.
- Select a breathing exercise that is comfortable, achievable and appropriate for your client. Create a craving, rate the craving and use the breathing exercise to help your client change state and reduce the intensity of the cravings.

BOX 10.9 Case study 4

Robert, aged 55 in remission from bladder cancer, reported feelings of 'not being able to cope'. His GP had diagnosed a panic disorder state and prescribed antidepressants. Robert was experiencing severe nicotine cravings and a feeling of 'burning rage'. Eye movement desensitization and reprocessing (EMDR) successfully neutralized the sensitizing events causing his panic attacks. Mindfulness 'easy breathing' techniques enabled Robert to observe and 'sit with' his feelings without being overwhelmed. Initial hypnotherapy sessions were aimed at building resilience and finding skilful ways of responding to his powerful emotions. Additionally, an aromastix was chosen to anchor powerful resource states of strength, self-soothing and courage. Robert reported after his sessions that he used the aromastix rather than 'having a fag' and it had helped him feel ready to stop smoking permanently and start 'living well'.

5. INSTALLING: NEW BEHAVIOURS, RESOURCES AND FEELINGS

Are you curious about how people become motivated to change or seek help to do so? Perhaps there has been an occasion in the past where you suddenly became absolutely fed-up about something in your life and you stopped doing things in the same way. Maybe you took a good look at yourself or someone or something and decided that things were going to change. In your personal life it can be interesting to note the similarities in these 'something's got to change' feelings and the strategies you use to accomplish those changes. This represents your personal 'blueprint' for change. However, each individual has a unique 'blueprint' that in turn reveals their locus of control and how their 'energy' for change is best utilized. Some individuals are motivated by driving away from the problem, e.g. 'I don't want to live in poverty'. While others are compelled 'towards' the solution, e.g. 'I create and welcome abundance'. It is important for the therapist to identify and match the client's most successful strategies for change but in the safety of the therapeutic space, what else may be possible? Invitations, experiments, creativity, curiosity, laughter, letting go of what no longer works and playfulness are just some suggestions to get you started.

Reflective practice 5

This practice is designed to help you identify compelling and powerful motivators to change. Once identified, they can be linked to resources and feelings that can support the desired behaviour (see Boxes 10.10 and 10.11).

6. NEGOTIATING: CONSCIOUS AND SUBCONSCIOUS OBJECTIONS TO CHANGE

Resistance and secondary gains are often mentioned as reasons why clients do not achieve their goals or sabotage their success. While these concepts can be useful to explore, they are strictly one-way and are directed only towards the client. It is also impossible for clients to refute such statements from their therapists. In neurolinguistic programming (NLP), resistance is a statement about what the therapist is doing rather than the client, and requires that the therapist becomes more flexible in the way they present themselves until they get a desired response. Such an approach certainly ensures that therapists take their share of responsibility for facilitating

Helping a person go Smoke Free: a reflective approach

BOX 10.10

Imagine if . . .
- Take a few moments to imagine you are a smoker. Notice what it feels like to label yourself in this way. Jot down possible reasons for stopping smoking. Make it real rather than spiel (sales talk). Which reasons are 'real' for you? How do you know the difference?

Finding something compulsive
- How could you identify which motivators are the most useful and compelling for your client and how could you amplify those feelings of motivation? How would you work with a client who prefers to keep his/her motivations very private?

Seek and you will find
- How could you identify and recreate resources that your client can generate and experience? How could you find resources that are outside of your client's conscious awareness or current behavioural experiences?

BOX 10.11 Case study 5

Alison, aged 62, with lung cancer, had smoked from 9 years and had never considered stopping. Scheduled for both radiotherapy and chemotherapy, Alison said 'there is no point in going through all that unless I stop'. On presentation, Alison was breathless and scored her cravings as 11/10, despite wearing a NRT patch. An initial breathing technique reduced this craving to 3/10.

Parts therapy without formal trance induction was used to establish two core self-beliefs of 'bloody minded' and 'independence'. The 'bloody minded' part (strong, right hand) decided it would stop smoking there and then. The 'independent' (left hand) refused to be told what to do by a cigarette and allied itself to 'bloody minded'. Thus, Alison held, within her two hands, all the resources needed to prevent a cigarette reaching her mouth.

This was reinforced in a subsequent trance session when the hypnotherapist underlined that any cravings would reactivate these resourceful parts. This craving control strategy was tested until an IMR signaled satisfaction. Future pacing of life as a non-smoker was sensitive to her acute health situation, and at Alison's specific request based on 'living life to the full while I can still breathe'. Alison was smoke free at the 12-week follow-up and reported being determined to remain smoke free.

change. Another approach is to simply view the lack of desired progress as an objection to change. The word objection implies an earnest and meaningful rationale behind the behaviour and invites both therapist and client to review and negotiate his/her smoking cessation aims.

Reflective practice 6

This practice is designed to help you consider issues that you and your client might experience when beginning change work. It also encourages the therapist to think outside of the box and be prepared to model optimism and flexibility (see Boxes 10.12 and 10.13).

BOX 10.12

Smoking 'but(s)'

■ How would you design a therapy session or intervention for a client who feels very unsure or undecided about stopping smoking?

Clearing the way for change

■ What are your thoughts about self-efficacy? How would you work with a client who you believe over/underestimates his/her self-efficacy?

Something came up

■ What therapeutic strategies would you use to support a client who is feeling increasingly depressed or despondent now that they have stopped smoking or felt that way in the past when they stopped?

Hannah, aged 57, was in remission from breast cancer and wished to stop smoking, as she was 'sick to death of being nagged about it' by her ex-smoker partner. Her two previous attempts at stopping had resulted in an extremely low mood and constant cravings. Hannah was fearful that she might experience depression again.

A contract was agreed to take non-smoking for a test drive in the imagination and find out how to 'get it right'. Hannah's session focused on connecting to her sense of core strength and her ability to decide for herself what she wanted to achieve. IMRs were installed to 'guard' her comfort and to signal if she felt discomfort. Hannah was future paced into 3 days as a non-smoker and invited to experience in her own time and way what that was like; what made a positive difference; what was less helpful and what strategies were surprisingly useful. Hannah emerged from her trance work feeling calm, content and willing to 'give it a go'.

Hannah returned 6 weeks later to inform her therapist that she had stopped but started smoking again. She felt very peaceful about her decision to start smoking and her partner's 'nagging' to quit, no longer upset her in the same way. The therapist thanked Hannah for her honesty and the privilege of working with her.

7. GATHERING: MOMENTUM AND DESIRE FOR A SMOKE-FREE FUTURE

This element of the SEEDING framework is one that can be revisited many times during a session either in formal eyes-closed processes or just a simple invitation to 'imagine'. It enables the therapist to calibrate their collaborative work and build a positive, realistic expectancy. Focusing on success, amplifying and reinforcing the positive steps your client is making and imagining what it would be like 'if . . .' are powerful change work tools that can energize the therapeutic relationship and promote self-efficacy. Pseudo-orientation in time (future pacing) can be used to rehearse non-smoking interventions and behaviours in potentially difficult trigger situations and permit a client to 'test-drive' what it feels like to be a non-smoker. It can also reveal any objections to a smoke-free lifestyle. These can be discussed and worked on consciously or the subconscious can take them to a deeper level to resolve any underlying conflicts or fine-tune plans. Maybe the subconscious would like to dream a bigger dream and use its power and resources to work on another project? Appropriate ego-strengthening and a carefully constructed metaphor relevant to the client (both techniques of course being relevant at any stage of the SEEDING framework) may be particularly helpful to nurture the client through the first behavioural changes and foster hope and resilience.

Reflective practice 7

This practice is designed to help you to calibrate to your client and select the most appropriate emotional tone and pace. The therapist is then invited to think 'what next' both for themselves and their clients (see Boxes 10.14 and 10.15).

BOX 10.14

Ready, steady, go . . .

■ How do you know when you have your client's conscious and subconscious consent to go for change? How could you recognize ambivalence or discomfort?

Bespoke suggestions

■ Are you comfortable with using stories, metaphor and examples from real-life scenarios? Take some time now to review the many ways in which you have been moved, entranced and inspired.

Time for a change

■ How do you feel about creating a silent space in your session to permit your client to find a personal and private moment away from your voice? How do you end your sessions with your client appropriately?

BOX 10.15 Case study 7

Dave, aged 26, a radiographer, requested help to stop his 20/day smoking behaviour. Dave's partner Sarah was due to give birth in 3 weeks time and he was 'excited' and 'worried' about becoming a father. His main motivation to stop was to save money and he chose to go 'cold turkey' and get it 'over with'.
In talking with Dave, he came to the realization that the cigarette that meant the most was the last one of the day, which provided a much needed quiet moment on the 'back door step'.

An 'aromastix' was created and Dave was encouraged to use the stick with a breathing technique and explore this private feelings. The therapist invited Dave to listen with a more powerful and profound part of his mind to a story about the single-mindedness and tenacity of babies as they grow and learn how to stand, toddle and walk. Using the technique of syntactical ambiguity, he was asked 'what else could he learn from a little baby' and invited to take some private, quiet time to 'consider what you are learning now' and 'how this could be used in the future'.

After several minutes of deep reflection Dave emerged refreshed and alert. After a single 80 min session, Dave remains a non-smoker.

CONCLUSION

Smoking cessation provides an ideal opportunity to demonstrate the effectiveness of hypnotherapy and its capacity to blend with and enhance the positive effects of other complementary therapies. Here we have briefly outlined just some of the synergistic possibilities of combining interventions. We hope to have created a desire for therapists to share expertise, integrate excellence from all therapy fields and develop new areas for research and investigation. In this chapter there are no 'lists' or step-by-step instructions/recommendations for practice, rather an acknowledgement that each client is unique and sessions can evolve from the integrity of the client/therapist relationship. In the tradition of Ericksonian hypnotherapy, experiential participation by the therapist and the creation of space for subconscious in-session reflection is recommended, indeed essential for shifting from rigidity to flow (Erickson & Rossi 1977). It is our belief that the shift for you is already happening.

REFERENCES

Ahijevych, K., Yerardi, R., Nedilsky, N., 2000. Descriptive outcomes of the American Lung Association of Ohio Hypnotherapy Smoking Cessation Program. Int. J. Clin. Exp. Hypn. 48 (4), 374–387.

Bala, M., Strzeszynski, L., Cahill, K., 2008. Mass media interventions for smoking cessation in adults. Cochrane Database Syst. Rev. (1), CD004704.

Erickson, M.H., Rossi, E.L., 1977. Autohypnotic experiences of Milton H. Erickson, MD. Am. J. Clin. Hypn. 20, 36–54. Reprinted in Rossi, E.L. (Ed.), 1980. The collected papers of M H Erickson, Vol. 1: The nature of hypnosis and suggestions. Irvington Press, New York.

Geary, B.B., 1994. Seeding responsiveness to hypnotic processes. In: Zeig, J.K. (Ed.), Ericksonian methods: the essence of the story. Brunner/Mazel, New York.

General Household Survey, 2006. Smoking and drinking in adults. Online. Available: www.statistics.gov.uk/downloads/ theme_compendia/GHS06/ Smokinganddrinkingamongadults2006. pdf.

Gibbs, G., 1988. Learning by doing: a guide to teaching and learning methods. Further Education Unit. Oxford Polytechnic (now Oxford Brookes University), Oxford.

Haley, J., 1973. Uncommon therapy: the psychiatric techniques of Milton H. Erickson. MD. Norton, New York.

Hernandez-Reif, M., Field, T., Hart, S., 1999. Smoking cravings are reduced by self-massage. Prev. Med. 28 (1), 29–31.

Johns, C., 2002. Guided reflection: advancing practice. Blackwell, Oxford.

Johns, C., 2004. Becoming a reflective practitioner, second ed. Blackwell, Oxford.

Lancaster, T., Stead, L., Silagy, C., et al., 2000. Effectiveness of interventions to help people stop smoking: findings from the Cochrane Library. Br. Med. J. 321 (7257), 355–358.

Maycock, P., Mackereth, P., 2009. Helping smokers to stop. The International Therapist 86, 18–19.

Morton-Cooper, A., Palmer, A., 2000. Mentoring, preceptorship and clinical supervision. Blackwell Science, Oxford.

Schön, D., 1983. The reflective practitioner – how professionals think in action. Arena, London.

Wellings, K., Macdowall, J.W., 2000. Evaluating mass media approaches to health promotion: a review of methods. Health Educ. 100 (1), 23–32.

White, A.R., Rampas, H., Ernst, E., 2000. Acupuncture for smoking cessation. Cochrane Database Syst. Rev. (2), CD000009.

Zeig, J.K., 1990. SEEDING. In: Zeig, J.K., Gilligan, S.G. (Eds.), Brief therapy: myths, methods and metaphors. Brunner/Mazel, New York.

FURTHER READING

DoH, 2004. Summary of intelligence on tobacco. Department of Health. HMSO, London.

DoH, 2008. Excellence in tobacco control: 10 high impact changes to achieve tobacco control. Department of Health, London. Online. Available: www.dh.gov.uk/ publication.

Hodkinson, Cook B, Mackereth, P., 2006. Creative approaches to reflexology. In: Mackereth, A., Carter, A. (Eds.), Massage and bodywork: adapting therapies for cancer care. Elsevier, London.

NICE, 2006. Brief interventions and referral for smoking cessation. National Institute for Clinical Excellence, London.

O'Hanlon, W.H., Martin, M., 1992. Solution-orientated hypnosis: an Ericksonian Approach. W W Norton, New York.

Zeig, J.K. (Ed.), 1985. Ericksonian psychotherapy, Vol. 1. Structures. Brunner/Mazel, New York.

Helping a person go Smoke Free: a reflective approach

USEFUL RESOURCES

The Christie NHS Foundation Trust, Wilmslow Rd, Withington, Manchester M20 4BX. Tel: 0161 446 8236 or e-mail: peter.mackereth@christie.nhs.uk.

NHS Stop Smoking Helpline: Tel: 0800 169 0 169 or website: www.gosmokefree.co.uk.

Pregnancy Smoking Helpline: Tel: 0800 169 9169 (12–9pm everyday).

NHS Asian Tobacco Helpline (1pm–9pm Tuesdays).

Urdu: Tel: 08001690881 (other language lines available).

The Milton H. Ericksonian Foundation, website: www.erickson-foundation.org/.

The Freedom From Smoking American. websitewww.ffsonline.org/.

Hypno-psychotherapy for adjustment and resilience in cancer care

Elizabeth Taylor

CHAPTER CONTENTS

CHAPTER OUTLINE

This chapter outlines the development and provision of a psychotherapeutic intervention to help patients cope with the diagnosis and treatment of cancer. Hypnotherapy and cognitive-behavioural therapy are combined in a clinical package, tailored to individual need. Despite some initial professional resistance to this approach, a qualitative study indicated a high level of satisfaction with the service. The findings also highlighted misconceptions about hypnotherapy and the need to provide a therapy setting sensitive to the needs of cancer patients undergoing active medical treatment. Participants' experiences of the programme are presented using extracts from this study. Demand for the service led to a multi-centre dissemination programme and the results are outlined. The chapter concludes with recommendations for training and development.

© 2010 Elsevier Ltd.
DOI: 10.1016/B978-0-7020-3082-6.00013-7

KEY WORDS

Cancer
Hypnotherapy
Cognitive-behavioural therapy
Dissemination project

INTRODUCTION

The diagnosis and treatment of cancer carries a heavy emotional burden, with approximately half of all cancer patients experiencing anxiety and depression severe enough to reach clinical significance. The National Institute for Clinical Excellence (NICE) (2004) recommends that routine psychological support should be available to all cancer patients and there is a substantial body of evidence demonstrating the efficacy of hypnotherapy and psychotherapy in cancer care. Psychological distress and morbidity are frequently reported following a cancer diagnosis and during active treatment (c.f. Zabora et al 2001). The latter can be further compounded by chemotherapy side-effects which can have a direct influence on appetite/ weight loss, muscular weakness, anxiety, depression and helplessness that, at worst, can affect treatment compliance (Walker et al 1999, Molassiotis et al 2002).

As nearly half of all cancer patients experience levels of anxiety and depression severe enough to affect their quality of life, NICE (2004) recommends that all patients should have access to psychological support. Historically this has been problematic, as health professionals were not trained to elicit patients' psychosocial concerns and focussed exclusively on the physical aspects of the disease. Patients' concerns therefore remained hidden and unresolved. The widespread training of senior health professionals in effective communication skills, however, has begun to redress the balance (Maguire & Pitceathley 2002, Fallowfield et al 2002, 2003, Wilkinson et al 2006). Even so, routine psychological support is not always available and some distressed cancer patients receive no psychological help at all (Greer et al 1997, Moorey & Greer 2002). These factors led REAL Wellbeing (a charitable organization in Northern England) to develop a psychotherapeutic intervention to help patients cope with the diagnosis and treatment of cancer. The intervention comprises effective elements of documented behavioural approaches in a clinical package to meet individual needs. Its official title is Psychological Support Services for Cancer Care but it is generally known as the 'hypno-chemo programme'. The latter is misleading because it implies that patients need to be receiving chemotherapy in order to access it. This is not the case and the programme is suitable for patients at all stages of the disease trajectory. Nevertheless, hypno-chemo has 'stuck' and become more meaningful to both patients and health professionals than the official term. The programme was developed during the period 1996–2000 from experience within the team and from studies demonstrating the efficacy of the approaches used, up to and during the initial development period. As such, it has been necessary to include a number of older references or seminal papers.

This chapter will describe the hypno-chemo programme, outlining the therapeutic content of hypnotherapy, relaxation training and cognitive-behavioural therapy (CBT). Selected research demonstrating the efficacy of these therapies is outlined alongside studies indicating the importance of involving patients in decision-making and provision of a psychologically supportive setting in cancer care. These include hypnotherapy and relaxation training to ameliorate the side-effects of chemotherapy. Relaxation training is used as an alternative to hypnotherapy when misconceptions about the latter cannot be overcome or there is a risk of adverse reaction to hypnosis. Evidence relating to the provision of CBT to reduce cancer-related psychological distress is addressed, followed by behavioural approaches for pain control. CBT is a talking therapy which identifies dysfunctional thinking and behaviours. The patient works towards cognitive restructuring and behavioural change. The priority for the selection of papers was that they needed to be relatively recent outcome studies (at the time), comparing one or more experimental conditions with at least one control group. These studies, however, are reported from a quantitative perspective, which restricts understanding of the individual patient's interpretation of events, and as a consequence, limits the opportunity to refine interventions more specifically to meet their needs. A post-intervention qualitative study was therefore conducted to separate out those elements of the hypno-chemo programme that most benefited participants, allowing their experiences to be fully assessed and viewed within the context of the situation (Taylor & Ingleton 2003). Patients' experiences from this study are presented, highlighting service satisfaction and areas requiring attention. The chapter concludes with a dissemination study and clinical audit to assess the feasibility of multi-centre service provision and recommendations for education, training and development.

THE HYPNO-CHEMO PROGRAMME

The hypno-chemo programme aims to provide adjuvant psychological support and has borrowed effective components from appropriate psychosocial interventions to develop a 12-session structured approach consisting of hypnotherapy and CBT. Hypnotherapy is used to teach relaxation, manage pain, prepare for and treat the side-effects of chemotherapy and facilitate guided imagery (GI) to give the patient a perceived tool with which to fight malignant cells. CBT is used to elicit and treat the emotional problems associated with cancer and treatment.

Requirements for inclusion are diagnosis of cancer at any stage and sufficient command of English (or other language common to both parties) to be able to work with the therapist. Patients with unstable psychotic illnesses are excluded, as the combination of therapies described is inappropriate in active psychosis, and their psychological treatment/medication is available through the usual NHS resources. Patients with stable psychotic illness can be accepted at the discretion of the therapist and with the agreement of the patient's psychiatrist. Hypnotherapy, however, is avoided with these patients and also in those diagnosed with malignant brain tumours to prevent any risk of adverse reaction.

ASSESSMENT

Patients are assessed and treated by the same psychotherapist. A medical history is taken, together with tumour histology, local/metastatic spread, medication and clinical treatment regimen. If pain management is required, a detailed sensory description of symptomatology is established. Psychosocial assessment aims to elicit patients' physical, social, psychological and spiritual concerns. The biological effects of chemotherapy and how conditioning exacerbates these are explained and reactions to previous or current chemotherapy identified. A simple explanation of immunology is given. The cognitive-behavioural model and hypnotic intervention are explained, concerns about hypnotherapy identified and a treatment plan agreed before written consent is obtained. Partners/carers are present at the initial consultation according to the patient's wishes.

HYPNOTHERAPY

Hypnosis is induced by eye fixation, passive muscle relaxation and appropriate deepening procedures (visualizing a peaceful scene, descending numbers, etc.). Treatment is tailored to individual need but typically involves relaxation, confidence-building suggestions and GI to deal with impending stressful procedures. Patients are taken verbally through the sequence of events leading to, during and following chemotherapy infusions. Occurring anxiety, nausea or other unpleasant sensations are cue-controlled by hypnotic suggestion. For example, the patient is asked to visualize a numerical dial representing nausea, and practise turning the dial up and down to obtain control. The latter is subsequently associated with a cue word, which is used to reduce nausea in the chemotherapy environment and with associated stimuli. Patients are asked to visualize their white blood cells attacking and destroying cancer cells using images/scenes of their choice. Pain modification is tailored to individual need. Imagery techniques are preferred for good hypnotic subjects (high hypnotizables), such as giving the pain a shape and colour and allowing it to float away. Distraction techniques are preferable for low hypnotizables, e.g. focussing on competing sensations elsewhere in the body such as rubbing the fingers together maintained by post-hypnotic suggestion. All procedures are supported by audio-taped instructions for daily practice and use during chemotherapy infusions if required.

Hypnotherapy is not always appropriate, as widespread misconceptions of involuntary mind control, perpetuated by the popular press and abuse by stage hypnotists, have led to fearful and sceptical beliefs. Most concerns are easily overcome by sensitive explanation and rapport but if patients cannot be reassured, progressive muscle relaxation (PMR) is used instead. This involves physical stretching and relaxing of consecutive muscles to induce relaxation, accompanied by visualization such as a peaceful scene and followed by cancer-related GI, as above. The need for PMR is minimal but unfortunately the active requirements of this technique can burden some already exhausted cancer patients.

CBT is used to identify and resolve cancer-related psychological problems and follows the procedures described by Greer et al (1992) and Greer (1997). This approach focuses on the personal meaning of cancer for the patient and the patient's coping strategies. Patients are encouraged to disclose and express the emotional impact of cancer on themselves and significant others, taught to identify the automatic dysfunctional thoughts underlying anxiety and depression, challenge these thoughts and replace them with more rational responses. Task-focussed behavioural assignments are encouraged to generate a sense of achievement and raise self-esteem. An attitude of reasonable optimism, determination not to give in, desire to understand and participate in treatment and continue to live a normal life is encouraged. This attitude characterizes 'fighting spirit' recommended by Greer and colleagues (1992). At REAL Wellbeing, this term is replaced by realistic positive thinking as recent evidence suggests patients can become burdened with guilt when they fail to maintain their fighting spirit (Watson et al 1999).

The combination of these approaches, tailored to individual needs represents the hypno-chemo programme, a popular intervention with demand surpassing resources. The psychosocial literature influencing the development and content of the programme is outlined below.

RESEARCH INFLUENCING THE DEVELOPMENT OF THE HYPNO-CHEMO PROGRAMME

Hypnotherapy and related procedures such as relaxation training and GI have been used to ameliorate the side-effects of chemotherapy, help patients adjust to the disease, counteract pain and anxiety and alter the mechanisms of immunity to hopefully improve prognosis. These interventions have been evaluated in a series of studies. Extensive reviews of this literature (e.g. Fawzy et al 1995) have concluded consistently that hypnotherapy is effective in the above areas, with the possible exception of enhancing survival. The randomized controlled trials (RCTs) relating to the latter have produced conflicting results with some limited by methodological flaws (Walker 1992, Fox 1995, 1998). Blake-Mortimer et al (1999) and Coyne et al (2007) provide a more recent debate on psychotherapy and cancer survival rates. However, quality, rather than quantity of life is the concern of the hypno-chemo programme and, although the methodology of some studies utilizing hypnotherapy has been criticized (c.f. Rajasekaran et al 2005), there is consistent empirical evidence to support the use and evaluation of this approach.

THE TREATMENT OF CHEMOTHERAPY SIDE-EFFECTS

HYPNOTHERAPY

The work of Walker and colleagues (1988) has been particularly influential in the development of the hypno-chemo programme and the cultivation of a professional but informal atmosphere at ELIHC. These researchers

Hypno-psychotherapy for adjustment and resilience in cancer care

developed an adjuvant approach to the treatment of chemotherapy side-effects using audio-recorded hypnotherapy with patients who, despite antiemetic medication, suffered severe side-effects. Anticipatory nausea was eliminated or improved in 88% of participants, all demonstrated improvement in treatment anxiety and all completed chemotherapy. Late-onset nausea/emesis was improved but not eliminated.

This approach was evaluated in a prospective RCT with 69 unselected patients with first diagnosis of Hodgkin's disease, non-Hodgkin's lymphoma or testicular teratoma, all undergoing first-line cytotoxic chemotherapy. Patients were randomly assigned to antiemetic drugs and relaxation, plus hypnotherapy or a control condition, which included discussion of side-effects and review of antiemetic regimen. A low incidence of side-effects overall, however, meant the study lacked statistical power. Nonetheless, results indicated that patients in the hypnotherapy condition had less treatment anxiety and patients in the relaxation condition had less late-onset nausea. The authors concluded that detailed explanation and concern about reducing side-effects may have had substantial prophylactic benefit (Walker et al 1992) supporting former research into the benefits of appropriate preparation for chemotherapy (Burish et al 1991).

This approach however, raises concerns about the use of audio-recorded hypnotic procedures in unselected patients. Adverse reactions can occur in a small minority (Finlay & Jones 1996) when traumatic, unconscious experiences are expressed. This cathartic release requires sensitive handling and the risk is greatly reduced by initial psychological assessment. Coping styles, known to influence optimal psychological intervention (Greer et al 1979, Pettingale 1984, Watson et al 1984) were not taken into account. Live relaxation training is generally superior to cassette recordings (Morrow 1984) and GI is more effective when provided by experienced therapists (Carey & Burish 1987). Nevertheless, Walker et al's results emphasize the necessity to provide detailed information and actively include patients in treatment regimens.

PROGRESSIVE MUSCLE RELAXATION

Building on the above findings, a rigorously conducted study has demonstrated that clinically significant distress need not be inevitable following diagnosis and during primary chemotherapy. Walker et al (1999) postulated that relaxation and GI would enhance response to adjuvant or neoadjuvant chemotherapy in addition to improved quality-of-life (QOL) and coping skills.

A total of 96 patients with newly diagnosed large or locally advanced breast cancer were randomized to receive standard care or standard care with PMR and GI (host defences destroying cancer cells). The groups did not differ significantly on medical or sociodemographic variables. A battery of psychometric tests was used to assess mood, QOL, personality and coping strategies. Mood and QOL was assessed before each of the 6 cycles of chemotherapy and 3 weeks after the final infusion. Personality and coping skills were examined prior to cycles 1 and 6. On completion of chemotherapy, clinical response rates were classified using the Standardized International

Union Against Cancer (UICC 1987) criteria and histological response assessed from excised breast tissue.

The intervention included PMR and cue-controlled relaxation, supported by audiotape. Cartoon pictures were issued to assist patients to visualize their host defences destroying malignant cells and daily practice was encouraged. Patients kept a diary to permit evaluation of technique practice, imagery vividness and response to chemotherapy. Daily practice compliance was high during the 18-week chemotherapy regimen. On completion, the intervention group demonstrated less psychological distress, less emotional suppression, increased relaxation and better QOL than controls. Although there were no differences in clinical or pathological responses to chemotherapy between the two groups, ratings of imagery vividness were positively correlated with degree of clinical response. Experimental patients had higher numbers of lymphokine-activated killer (LAK) cell cytotoxicity, activated T-cells and reduced blood levels of tumour necrosis factor. The authors are unclear about the clinical significance of these enhanced immunological effects in the light of their results.

One important finding was the low incidence of clinically significant mood disturbance in both groups (4% before and 2% after chemotherapy). This was attributed to the setting that provides open access for patients and carers. Staff are sensitive to the need for information and advice, actively elicit and deal with concerns and include patients in treatment decisions if they wish. Waiting times for chemotherapy are minimized. A post-treatment satisfaction audit indicated that 93% of both groups were 'satisfied/very satisfied' with the psychological support provided, and attrition was minimal. The authors conclude that routine psychological support is superior to the more usual specialist service, which treats emotional problems only when they have reached clinical significance.

COGNITIVE-BEHAVIOUR THERAPY FOR CANCER-RELATED PSYCHOLOGICAL DISTRESS

The work of Greer et al (1992) has strongly influenced the hypno-chemo programme. These workers conducted a controlled trial to determine the efficacy of Adjuvant Psychological Therapy (APT), a CBT approach specifically designed for cancer care. Patients with primary diagnosis or first recurrence of mixed cancers were screened for psychological morbidity using the Hospital Anxiety and Depression (HAD) scale (Zigmond & Snaith 1983) and the Mental Adjustment to Cancer (MAC) scales (Greer & Watson 1987, Watson et al 1988). The latter measures four broad dimensions of adjustment: fighting spirit, helplessness, anxious preoccupation and fatalism. A total of 174 patients with scores above previously defined cut-off points were randomly assigned to experimental or control conditions. Experimental patients individually participated in the 8-week, problem-focussed APT programme, while controls received no therapy. Outcome measures included the HAD and MAC scales, Rotterdam Symptom Check List (RSC, De Haes et al 1990) and the Psychosocial Adjustment to Illness Scale (Derogatis 1983). The trial was completed by 90% of patients.

The intervention, which aimed to detect and treat the emotional problems associated with the disease included cognitive restructuring, behavioural assignments, PMR and role-play/imagination to deal with imminent stressful procedures. Immediately following the intervention, the therapy group had significantly lower scores on helplessness, anxious preoccupation and fatalism, anxiety, psychological symptoms and orientation to healthcare, and significantly higher scores on fighting spirit than controls. At the 4-month follow-up, experimental patients continued to have significantly lower scores on anxiety and psychological symptoms/distress. At the 12-month follow-up (Moorey et al 1994) patients who had received therapy still had less anxiety and depression than controls. The authors concluded that APT significantly reduces cancer-related psychological morbidity, thus enhancing the psychological dimension of QOL. However, one-third of eligible patients refused to take part and the author did not report any adverse therapy effects. No post-intervention qualitative assessment was conducted to indicate in detail which elements of the intervention the participants valued the most.

BEHAVIOURAL APPROACHES IN THE MANAGEMENT OF PAIN

Adjuvant pain management is an important component in the hypno-chemo programme, which may be cancer, treatment-related, or general pain. There is substantial literature on the use of hypnotherapy in the management of pain but some workers suggest CBT is also effective in management. The manifestation of pain is predictable in bone marrow transplantation (BMT) providing an opportunity to test the efficacy of psychosocial interventions.

Syrjala et al (1992) postulated that both hypnosis and CBT would reduce treatment-related pain in this group of adults. Prior to their first transplantation, 67 BMT patients with haematological malignancies were randomized to one of four groups: hypnotherapy, CBT, therapist contact control or treatment as usual. Age, gender and a risk variable, based on diagnosis and relapse/remission rates, comprised biodemographic data. Physical functioning was assessed by the Sickness Impact Profile (SIP, Bergner et al 1976, 1981) with daily records of pain and nausea monitored on a visual analogue scale (VAS). Psychological symptoms were addressed by the Brief Symptom Inventory (BSI, Derogatis & Spencer 1982) and psychologist assessment. The SIP and BSI were used as covariates in the analysis. The intervention and therapist contact groups met with a clinical psychologist for 2×90 min sessions prior to transplant and 10×30 min reinforcement sessions after in-patient admission. Hypnotherapy consisted of relaxation and imagery targeted towards the reduction of pain and nausea and emotional reactions to the latter, together with suggestions of enhanced coping/control and well-being. Audio-taped instructions for daily practise were issued. CBT consisted of education about the mechanisms of pain and nausea with the benefits of reducing physiological arousal, together with cognitive restructuring, coping strategies, goal setting and PMR. The therapist contact condition included general discussion with no introduction of new coping skills. In the treatment as usual group, patients received standard medical care only. The remaining 45 patients provided covariate and time series data.

Results indicated that the hypnotic intervention only, was effective in reducing treatment-related pain. There were no significant differences in nausea, emesis and opioid use between the treatment groups and, contrary to expectations, CBT did not ameliorate the symptoms measured. The authors emphasize the importance of imagery in such interventions. This was not included in the CBT group and patients intermittently refused sessions with relaxation alone when treatment stress shortened attention span. During this stage, hypnotherapy patients also preferred shortened inductions/relaxation routines and more engaging imagery. Although the authors conducted no qualitative evaluation, they suggest the impact of both interventions on nausea and vomiting may be limited by inadequate training. Rather than a gradual onset, the first dose of chemotherapy produced severe emesis, which prevented the practise opportunities afforded to other cancer populations. This, coupled with cognitive side-effects of high-dose antiemetics and opioids, may have been too great a challenge to a newly learnt skill. The study only measured symptom intensity and the small sample size may have had inadequate power to demonstrate efficacy in all variables measured. Methods of pain and nausea control were not made clear, making replication difficult. Nevertheless, the study demonstrates the superiority of hypnotherapy and GI in pain management supporting a former large-scale RCT with 109 metastatic breast cancer patients. In their seminal paper, Spiegal and Bloom (1983) concluded that supportive group therapy coupled with hypnosis provided greater pain control than supportive therapy alone.

To obtain an in-depth insight and understanding of participant experience, a qualitative enquiry was conducted. Eight patients who had completed the hypno-chemo programme were purposefully selected. Seven had breast cancer and one had colon cancer at the stage of local disease or local disease and regional spread. All underwent surgery and chemotherapy and seven received radiotherapy. Six patients commenced therapy just before or after their first session of chemotherapy. One patient joined the programme approximately halfway through chemotherapy and another after the latter was completed. Semi-structured interviews were conducted between 1 and 24 months (average 7 months) after the intervention and transcribed verbatim for thematic analysis. Primary themes identified were: gaining help, treatment tailored to needs, long-term benefits and service satisfaction/information needs. The findings demonstrated that participants had acquired advanced skills to enable them to cope, both with invasive medical procedures and with the psychological traumas they faced. The study also indicated difficulties in accessing the service, initial misconceptions about hypnotherapy and the need to provide a therapy setting sensitive to the needs of cancer patients undergoing active medical treatment. Extracts from the study illustrate patients' experiences.

Hypno-psychotherapy for adjustment and resilience in cancer care

There was an initial reluctance for health professionals to refer, possibly due to misconceptions about hypnosis and the low priority given to psychological concerns at that time (Taylor et al 2004). Typical quotations illustrate:

I was desperate to talk to someone but I was halfway through my chemo before I heard about it, nobody mentioned it before September; I started my chemo in May. If I hadn't been so poorly, I doubt that she would have mentioned it, you know . . . . I was so well after the . . . hypnotherapy, that if I'd had it at the beginning, I feel it would have been a lot, lot better, but nobody mentioned anything.

(Doreen)

I was talking to the nurse about my desire to go to . . . the cancer centre at Bristol . . . I couldn't go because the dates just didn't fit in with my treatment. . . . I felt it would be helpful for me to feel I was doing something positive. I said, is there nothing in this area? And very reluctantly I was told, well you could go to East Lancs (REAL Wellbeing) and I was so thrilled.

(Joyce)

Fear of chemotherapy was paramount and this, coupled with feeling overwhelmed by their diagnosis, led some patients to grasp the hypno-chemo programme as a lifeline. Exemplified below:

When I got the letter and leaflets telling me about the side-effects of chemotherapy, I was absolutely terrified. I went in trembling with fear.

(Joyce)

. . . you feel absolutely helpless and hopeless and . . . you can't influence anything in your life.

(Jenny)

All participants received hypnotherapy, however, many had negative preconceived beliefs and assumed they would lose consciousness or relinquish control to the therapist. For example:

I could only picture the non-clinical hypnosis; the stage stuff and I didn't really know what it was.

(Brenda)

Some patients were inhibited from attending the centre because it was next door to a hospice, illustrated below:

Well the first thought is. Oh no, the hospice. Why? Do they think I'm going to die?

(Jenny)

This 'one way ticket' was a common belief, with patients recommending a separate building off site.

All participants said they would recommend the service to others. For example:

I was so thrilled with it I felt I [laughs] wanted to help promote it so, so I actually took leaflets and they're there in the clinic after I'd taken them.

(Joyce)

This theme has implications for information giving, referral procedures and the provision of an appropriate environment, supporting the work of Walker and colleagues (1992).

TREATMENT TAILORED TO INDIVIDUAL NEEDS

This theme represents the identification of patients' main concerns and adopting appropriate therapies to aid their resolution. Following the patient's agenda rather than the therapist's is illustrated by the following quote:

They obviously try to assess exactly what your personal needs are and try to work to them.

(Christine)

Not only was this appreciated but patients also valued the therapists themselves. Given that the latter is recognized as an important variable in treatment outcome, it was noteworthy to discover that all participants considered the therapist as skilful and important in their adjustment to their various situations. For example:

She is obviously very, very talented.

(Christine)

I couldn't have managed without her ... I leant on her an awful lot and I could just go in and say, right, you want to know what's gone wrong now? Because I've had a few sort of family crises as well ... she just let me carry on ... that was the biggest part of it ... actually being able to talk.

(Susan)

Sharing personal problems was important for many patients:

My personal problem was the end of the world and [cries] it was far more grievous and stress causing than the cancer was. ... I ... welcomed the opportunity to share it with someone who I wasn't related to, or go to church with, and people who would undoubtedly be quite distressed by some of the things I had to say.

(Beryl)

Even if it ... hurts a bit ... I think you have to talk to somebody because I think it's too much for anyone to just, to cope ... and keep it to themselves.

(Brenda)

Understanding the cognitive model and utilizing the techniques within it are considered essential to the efficacy of CBT (Bottomley 1998). However, rather than demonstrating comprehension of the model and separating out the cognitive and behavioural elements, participants tended to view the intervention as a package. A typical vignette illustrates how patients amalgamated CBT with hypnotherapeutic aspects and GI in their understanding of altered thoughts and enhanced control.

I thought I was going to be as sick as anything for 6 months, that was the thing that was frightening me ... I think it made me feel more in control because that's why I was so upset in the beginning because I felt that I'd no control over what was happening ... I wasn't a relaxed person before it all started. I was sort of a very busy person and found it hard to switch off and I think it was good ... the fact that I was given a tool whereby I could switch off the nausea ... I did what I was told and I think I could always hear [named therapist's] voice [laughs] er ... telling me what to do.

(Patricia)

Some patients commented on their improvement without reference to specific techniques. For example:

I think it makes you have a different view of things ... it just helped somehow or other ... you weren't so uptight if people asked you anything, you weren't like drawing in on yourself or bursting out in tears or whatever, you just took it, you know, as it came.

(Brenda)

The exception to this was relaxation. Patients were very clear on how relaxation helped them particularly with sleep disturbance, chemotherapy and pain management. Typical vignettes illustrate:

I had real problems sleeping all the way through my treatment and ... [named therapist] gave me ... a sleep tape as well, which really, really helped er ... and the relaxation helped. I took it down to my chemotherapy sessions and for the couple of days afterwards when I felt particularly bad, er ... I used to play the tapes a few times a day and they really, really did help.

(Christine)

I think my pain I was in ... a lot of it, was lack of being relaxed ... I think psychical pain is caused by real tension or worry ... pain all over ... and I've never felt so relaxed in my life ....

(Jenny)

The latter provides a good example of holistic pain management and the need for multidimensional assessment (Davies & McVicar 2000), in this case, the patient's perception of pain. Jenny accurately described her chronic pain as a maladaptive fight, flight response, eloquently explained by Wall (1999). The body's attention to pain is observed as a state of alertness, including muscle tension, stiffness, disturbed sleep, alert immune system and lethargic gut. The longer this state continues the more anxiety is felt, leading to reduced pain tolerance and increased pain intensity. As Jenny put it, 'pain all over'. Jenny's pain was successfully treated by hypnotherapy, which taught her how to relax tense muscles, distract her attention and promote sleep.

A technique referred to as vein enlargement is used at ELIHCC, simply conducted by hypnotherapy and GI. A typical script demonstrates the technique:

'Visualize your veins as full swollen rivers; see the needle go firmly into the vein, let the vein and skin wrap themselves tightly around the needle so there is no leakage, no discomfort etc.'

This approach was greatly appreciated, e.g.

I was ... frightened of chemotherapy, because I've got bad veins ... my hands used to swell, my arms ... chemotherapy was terrible. I used to dread going in, but it never bothered me after she gave me a session on it, it pumped my veins up.

(Doreen)

No empirical research about this technique was revealed in the literature search. However, anecdotal reports support the use of this strategy in cancer care (Hammond 1990).

Feeling in control, confidence building and the visualization of host defences destroying cancer cells complete this theme and are closely inter woven. The need for control over what was happening to patients was an important finding with the 'cancer cell attack' considered a principal tool:

I wanted to fight this thing with whatever I could get.

(Joyce)

I think a person has to feel that they can do something about it.

(Jenny)

It was commented on at the hospital that I'd got the [laughs] the most positive attitude that they'd encountered .... I have stopped feeling such a victim and I have learnt some more strategies for coping with things.

(Beryl)

This attitude supports research recommending the controversial topic of fighting spirit (Greer et al 1992). Nevertheless, feeling part of the clinical team was necessary to patients, as illustrated below:

I think it really helped me relax all the way through and visualizing that I was actually helping my body to get rid of the cancer and make myself better.

(Christine)

The combination of techniques was considered to reduce helplessness and subsequent anxiety leading to an increase in confidence. For example:

I definitely lost confidence in myself. I think in the beginning ... but I feel as though [laughs] I've become a lot more confident probably than I was before, a lot more daring than I used to be and I'll say what I think to whom I think.

(Patricia)

If you're confident and happy in yourself then ... you can cope with things a lot better than if you were in an anxious state.

(Joyce)

These findings support a substantial body of evidence demonstrating the efficacy of behavioural approaches in cancer care. For example, in a review of psychosocial interventions at varying stages of disease, specific and heterogeneous cancers and including some large-scale RCTs, Fawzy et al (1995) found psychological and physiological improvements together with enhanced immune functioning for studies utilizing behaviour/cognitive-behaviour therapy. The consistency of positive outcomes in this area (Greer et al 1992, Walker 1992) highlights the desirability of their transference into routine clinical provision.

LONG-TERM BENEFITS

Patients continued to benefit from the techniques learned after discharge. One patient, interviewed 8 months after completion of chemotherapy said:

Hypno-psychotherapy for adjustment and resilience in cancer care

I'm still using the techniques I was taught ... I had my kitchen replaced ... and I got thoroughly stressed out. I thought you're going to give yourself cancer back again because you're worrying so much, so I listened to the cancer cell attack ... and it was a great help because I got the kitchen done ... without having to feel totally stressed out.

(Beryl)

Others used their learned skills to reduce tension and aid sleep. The use of cue-controlled GI is illustrated below:

You know, that's happened in the past or whatever ... then you cross your fingers and every time you cross your fingers you'll think of that scene ... I have used that such a lot afterwards for relaxation if I'm tense.

(Jenny)

Patients found they were able to relax at will:

If I wake up and I can't sleep I start relaxing my body.

(Susan)

Patients were able to express their feelings more openly. One patient interviewed after 2 years demonstrated this ability:

The difference now of course is that I've made friends with fellow cancer sufferers and that we do talk very, very honestly ... which I hadn't got before, I hadn't got anybody.

(Patricia)

These findings again support outcome studies utilizing CBT and hypnotherapy. In Greer and colleagues' study (1992), patients who had received APT continued to have significantly lower scores on anxiety and depression than controls at 12-month follow-up (Moorey et al 1994). Spiegal et al's (1981) early controversial work on hypno-psychotherapy and survival, demonstrated superior psychological health in experimental patients compared to controls at 10-year follow-up. Similar benefits have been demonstrated in patients with malignant melanoma (Fawzy et al 1993) and Hodgkin's/non-Hodgkin's lymphoma (Ratcliffe et al 1995).

Both this and the previous theme clearly demonstrate that patients need to feel in control of their situation and enhance their immunology. This was true for all participants and, providing the cancer cell approach is offered honestly and ethically, that is without inappropriate reassurance or raising false hopes, it appears to be a valuable technique depending on disease stage and patient choice.

SERVICE IMPROVEMENTS

This theme focuses on service satisfaction and identifies areas for improvement. Patients invariably viewed their therapy positively. The main criticism was lack of information about the existence of the service in appropriate clinics, closely followed by the need for health professionals to explain the programme beforehand. For example:

It's wonderful ... well it was just absolutely a Godsend to me because er ... struggling on my own, the thought of coming and having that hour with [named therapist].

(Joyce)

There is nothing I found that I thought could be improved other than it was at Rossendale, three buses away.

(Beryl)

Apart from [named breast care nurse] mentioning it, I didn't even know it existed.

(Christine)

Future availability was a major finding with most patients suggesting follow-up sessions or later treatment on request.

There was, however, evidence of service dissatisfaction related to medical procedures. Despite the widely publicized move from closed to open awareness, communication deficits were apparent.

... and they sent me down for a scan and they found my cancer, but they didn't mention cancer. They just said ... we'll have to operate on your bowels ... and somebody just ... threw me a paper in at the door and ... she said, er ... that's to do with your bag [colostomy]. Well it ... never registered ... and I have to have a bag and she left me... I was terrified then.

(Doreen)

Some patients complained about hospital waiting times, mechanical failure and human error, illustrated below:

Oh the waiting there was a nightmare ... They'd say, oh there's been a fault in the machine or I'm sorry your prescription should have been ordered last week and it hasn't and ... you were trapped there, you couldn't go home because you'd not had your chemo, you know, you'd wait for your bloods, you'd wait for your treatment.

(Susan)

Others were upset by the methods of breaking bad news and treatment delays, illustrated below:

I got a phone call ... no questions about who was with me, what I was doing. So, you've got cancer ... So I felt that was very bad and I felt the fact that it was 10 weeks before I went to theatre was absolutely dreadful.

(Joyce)

Collectively, the findings highlight the need for open communication, identification of concerns, information provision, and interventions tailored to individual need. Effective communication is central to all these issues and much is currently being done to address deficits in the wider palliative care community by the requirement for widespread training in Advanced Communications in Cancer Care (National Cancer Action Team 2008).

The high level of service satisfaction with the hypno-chemo programme greatly increased referrals, and demand for the service highlighted the need for teaching and dissemination. Therefore, the feasibility of clinical provision in wider England was assessed by conducting an audit of the

Hypno-psychotherapy for adjustment and resilience in cancer care

quality of training and service delivery, together with a cost analysis (Taylor et al 2006). Organizational approval was obtained from 36 palliative care centres.

A range of audit standards were monitored relating to the target population of patients, therapists, palliative care teams, tutors and supervisors. The method of data collection was the hard copy of audit tools and a range of analyses were conducted based on descriptive statistics.

All therapists attending the course met the pre-course requirements in relation to qualifications, insurance and membership of a professional organization. All prospective palliative care teams were sent the relevant information packs within the agreed time of 15 working days. The 36 therapists who completed the course in full all successfully met the training criteria. Response times for contacting the patient within 7 working days of receiving the referral was met 94% of the time and for making assessment appointments within 15 working days was met on 92% of occasions. All therapist records regarding patient appointments, supervision and pay claims were received in office each month with all essential documentation enclosed. Monthly, quarterly and twice-yearly supervision requirements were met by all therapists. Evaluation forms from the five key stakeholders (patients, therapists, palliative care teams, tutors and supervisors) showed positive attitudes towards the structure and running of the programme.

A total of 1244 patients were treated over the 2-year period with a large female majority. There was a wide age range of 18–89 years with an average age of 54. A total of 44 primary cancer sites were identified, with breast cancer accounting for approximately half of the sample. Patient outcomes indicated a high percentage of symptom relief pre- to post-treatment. The mean number of sessions for patients reporting elimination of their symptoms was 10, suggesting this is the optimal number of sessions required for patients receptive to techniques taught on the programme. Despite problems with integrating therapists in established workforces in some centres and a slow start in year 1 of the study, the success of the hypno-chemo programme was demonstrated as audit standards were consistently met and user views were for the most part positive.

Grant funding for service provision ceased in November 2005 and there was much concern from palliative care centres about the service ending. The programme supports one of the main aims of the NHS Cancer Plan (DoH 2000) to ensure that communication, information provision, psychological support, patient empowerment and palliative care are improved to reduce inequalities in service provision. Therefore, ways to sustain delivery remain important. Analysis of costs indicated value for money and every effort was made to assist participating centres to source continuation funding. This was problematic with the significant debt reported by the NHS at the time. However, 55% of centres were able to retain their therapist. The information obtained from the 3-year study was used to inform the purchasers and providers of cancer care and it was anticipated that the project might encourage primary care trusts to commission service provision.

SUMMARY

This chapter has outlined the development and clinical provision of combined hypnotherapy and cognitive-behavioural therapy in cancer care. Published work in areas of principal importance has been discussed. A qualitative investigation supporting these findings has added further insights to the patients' experience, which is not always possible using quantitative methods of enquiry. Patients were able to describe how hypnotherapy and CBT had helped them to cope with the diagnosis and treatment of cancer, with learned skills considered valuable tools in rehabilitation or remission. Participants would have preferred to undergo therapy in a hospital-based cancer unit or standalone setting rather than adjacent to a hospice. Conversely, some dissatisfaction was expressed with the hospital-based procedure. Participants were keen to recommend the hypno-chemo programme but were concerned about lack of information about the service. Including health professionals in a multi-centre study, however, has done much to overcome their mistrust of hypnotherapy and initial reluctance to support the programme. Indeed, a substantial number retained their therapist on cessation of funding. One important finding from the multi-centre study was that 10, rather than 12 sessions, were sufficient for a successful outcome, which reduced costs.

RECOMMENDATIONS FOR TRAINING AND DEVELOPMENT

Although 55% of participating centres continued to fund the hypno-chemo programme on cessation of grant funding, demand for the service has generated waiting lists with some patients having completed chemotherapy before being seen. This unacceptable situation is incongruent with NICE (2004) guidance and, as there has been no financial support from Primary Care Trusts, ways need to be found to generate income for this popular intervention. Subject to funding, the programme is available for national dissemination. Alternatively, training could be provided for appropriately qualified personnel. A further suggestion is to provide a continuum of evidence by conducting a phase 2 and phase 3 RCT, thus enhancing the possibility of mainstream funding. This may be an appropriate course of action for an interested graduate working towards a higher degree.

AWARDS

The hypno-chemo programme has won two awards:

- The Community in Action Award (2005) for the greatest contribution to Rossendale, Lancashire (Winner)
- The Prince of Wales Foundation for Integrated Health (2006) for the year 1 evaluation of the multi-centre study (Runner up).

ACKNOWLEDGEMENTS

We are grateful to the BIG Lottery for supporting the multi-centre study and to the research participants.

Hypno-psychotherapy for adjustment and resilience in cancer care

Bergner, M., Bobitt, R.A., Pollard, W.E., et al., 1976. The Sickness Impact Profile: validation of a health-status measure. Med. Care 14, 57–67.

Bergner, M., Bobitt, R.A., Carter, W.B., et al., 1981. The Sickness Impact Profile: development and final revision of a health-status measure. Med. Care 21, 787–805.

Blake-Mortimer, J., Gore-Felton, C., Kimerling, J.M., et al., 1999. Improving the quality and quantity of life among patients with cancer: a review of the effectiveness of group psychotherapy. Eur. J. Cancer 35 (11), 1581–1586.

Bottomley, A., 1998. Group cognitive behavioural therapy with cancer patients: the views of women participants on a short-term intervention. Eur. J. Cancer Care (Engl) 7, 23–30.

Burish, T.G., Snyder, S.L., Jenkins, R.A., 1991. Preparing patients for cancer chemotherapy: effective coping preparation and relaxation interventions. J. Consult. Clin. Psychol. 59, 518–525.

Carey, M.P., Burish, T.G., 1987. Providing relaxation training to cancer chemotherapy patients: a comparison of three delivery techniques. J. Consult. Clin. Psychol. 55, 732–737.

Coyne, J.C., Stefanek, M., Palmer, S.C., 2007. Psychotherapy and survival in cancer: the conflict between hope and evidence. Psychol. Bull. 133 (3), 367–394.

Davies, J., McVicar, A., 2000. Issues in effective pain control 2: from assessment to management. Int. J. Palliat. Nurs. 6 (4), 162–169.

De Haes, J.C., Van Knippenberg, F.C., Niejt, J.P., 1990. Measuring psychological and physical distress in cancer patients: structure and application of the Rotterdam Symptom Check List. Br. J. Cancer 62, 1034–1038.

Derogatis, L.R., Spencer, P.M., 1982. Brief Symptom Inventory (BSI) administration and procedures: BSI manual. John Hopkins University, Baltimore.

Derogatis, L.R., Morrow, G.R., Fetting, J., 1983. The prevalence of psychiatric disorders among cancer patients. J. Am. Med. Assoc. 249, 751–757.

DoH, 2000. The NHS Cancer Plan. Department of Health, London.

Fallowfield, L., Jenkins, V., Farewell, V., et al., 2002. Efficacy of a cancer research UK communication skills training model for oncologists: a randomised controlled study. Lancet 359 (9307), 650–656.

Fallowfield, L., Jenkins, V., Farewell, V., et al., 2003. Enduring impact of communication skills training. Results of a 2-month follow-up. Br. J. Cancer 89, 1445–1449.

Fawzy, F.I., Fawzy, N.W., Hyun, C.S., et al., 1993. Malignant melanoma: effects of an early structured psychiatric intervention, coping and affective state on recurrence and survival 6 years later. Arch. Gen. Psychiatry 50, 681–689.

Fawzy, F.I., Fawzy, N.W., Arndt, L.A., et al., 1995. Critical review of psychosocial interventions in cancer care. Arch. Gen. Psychiatry 52, 100–113.

Finlay, I.G., Jones, O.L., 1996. Hypnotherapy in palliative care. J. R. Soc. Med. 89, 493–496.

Fox, B.H., 1995. Some problems and some solutions in research on psychotherapeutic interventions in cancer. Support. Care Cancer 3, 257–263.

Fox, B.H., 1998. A hypothesis about Spiegel et al's 1989 paper on psychosocial intervention and breast cancer survival. Psychooncology 7, 361–370.

Greer, S., Watson, M., 1987. Mental adjustment to cancer: its measurement and prognostic significance. Cancer Surv. 6, 439–453.

Greer, S., 1997. Adjunctive psychological therapy for cancer patients. Palliat. Med. 11, 240–244.

Greer, S., Morris, T., Pettingale, K.W., 1979. Psychological response to breast cancer: effect on outcome. Lancet ii, 785–787.

Greer, S., Moorey, S., Baruch, D.R., et al., 1992. Adjuvant psychological therapy for patients with cancer: a prospective randomised trial. Br. Med. J. 304, 675–680.

Hammond, D.C., 1990. Handbook of hypnotic suggestions and metaphors. Norton, London.

Maguire, P., Pitceathley, C., 2002. Key communication skills and how to acquire them. Br. Med. J. 325, 697–700.

Molassiotis, A., Yung, H.P., Yam, B.M., et al., 2002. The effectiveness of progressive muscle relaxation training in managing chemotherapy-induced nausea

APPROACHES IN CLINICAL PRACTICE

and vomiting in Chinese breast cancer patients: a randomised controlled trial. Support. Care Cancer 10 (3), 237–246.

Moorey, S., Greer, S., 2002. Cognitive behaviour therapy for people with cancer. Oxford University Press, Oxford.

Moorey, S., Greer, S., Watson, M., et al., 1994. Adjuvant psychological therapy for patients with cancer: outcome at one year. Psychooncology 3, 39–46.

Morrow, G.R., 1984. Appropriateness of taped versus live relaxation in the systematic desensitization of anticipatory nausea and vomiting in cancer patients. J. Consult. Clin. Psychol. 52, 1098–1099.

National Cancer Action Team, 2008. National Advanced Communication Skills Training Programme for senior health professionals in cancer care. London Strategic Health Authority, London.

National Institute for Clinical Excellence (NICE), 2004. Improving supportive and palliative care for adults with cancer. Department of Health, London.

Pettingale, K.W., 1984. Coping and cancer prognosis. J. Psychosom. Res. 28, 363–364.

Rajasekaran, M., Edmonds, P.M., Higginson, I.L., 2005. Systematic review of hypnotherapy for treating symptoms in terminal ill adult cancer patients. Palliat. Med. 19, 418–426.

Ratcliffe, M.A., Dawson, A.A., Walker, L.G., 1995. Eysenck personality inventory L-Scores in patients with Hodgkin's disease and non-Hodgkin's lymphoma. Psychooncology 4, 39–45.

Spiegal, D., Bloom, J.R., 1983. Group therapy and hypnosis reduce metastatic breast carcinoma pain. Psychosom. Med. 45, 333–339.

Spiegal, D., Bloom, J.R., Yalom, I., 1981. Group support for patients with metastatic breast cancer. Arch. Gen. Psychiatry 38, 527–533.

Syrjala, K.L., Cummings, C., Donaldson, G.W., 1992. Hypnosis or cognitive behavioural training for the reduction of pain and nausea during cancer treatment: a controlled trial. Pain 48, 137–146.

Taylor, E.E., Ingleton, C., 2003. Hypnotherapy and cognitive-behaviour therapy in cancer care: the patients' view. Eur. J. Cancer Care (Engl) 12, 137–142.

Taylor, E.E., Ismail, S., Hills, H.M., et al., 2004. Multicomponent psychosocial support for newly diagnosed cancer patients: participants' views. Int. J. Palliat. Nurs. 10 (6), 287–295.

Taylor, E.E., Hills, H.M., Butterworth, C.J., et al., 2006. A multi-centre feasibility study and clinical audit of hypnotherapy and cognitive-behaviour therapy in cancer care. Unpublished report. Available on request from: liz.taylor@realtd.co.uk. East Lancashire Integrated Health Care.

UICC [International Union Against Cancer], 1987. TNM classification of malignant tumours. UICC, Berlin.

Walker, L.G., 1992. Hypnosis with cancer patients. American Journal of Preventative Psychiatry and Neurology 3 (3), 42–49.

Walker, L.G., Dawson, A.A., Ratcliffe, M.A., et al., 1988. Sick to death of it: psychological aspects of cytotoxic chemotherapy side-effects. Aberdeen Postgraduate Medical Bulletin 22, 11–17.

Walker, L.G., Walker, M.B., Ogston, K., et al., 1999. Psychological, clinical and pathological effects of relaxation training and guided imagery during primary chemotherapy. Br. J. Cancer 80 (1/2), 262–268.

Wall, P., 1999. Pain: The science of suffering. Weidenfield and Nicholson, London.

Watson, M., Greer, S., Blake, S., et al., 1984. Reaction to a diagnosis of breast cancer: relationship between denial, delay and rates of psychological morbidity. Cancer 53 (3), 2008–2012.

Watson, M., Greer, S., Young, J., et al., 1988. Development of a questionnaire measure of adjustment to cancer: the MAC scale. Psychol. Med. 18, 203–209.

Watson, M., Haviland, J.S., Greer, S., et al., 1999. Influence of psychological response on survival in breast cancer: a population-based cohort study. Lancet 354, 1331–1336.

Wilkinson, S.M., Perry, R., Linsell, L., et al., 2006. A randomized controlled trial to evaluate the efficacy of a three-day communication skills training programme for palliative care nurses. Palliat. Med. 20 (2), 139.

Zabora, J., BrintzenhofeSzoc, K., Curbow, B., et al., 2001. The prevalence of psychological distress by cancer site. Psychooncology 10 (1), 19–28.

Zigmond, A.S., Snaith, R.T., 1983. The hospital anxiety and depression scale. Acta Psychiatr. Scand. 67, 361–370.

Hypno-psychotherapy for adjustment and resilience in cancer care

REAL Wellbeing, St James Centre, 8 St James Square, Bacup, Lancashire OL13 9AA. Tel: 01706 871730; e-mail: info@realtd.co.uk; website: www.realltd.co.uk.

The National Register of Hypnotherapists and Psychotherapists, First Floor, 18 Carr Road, Nelson, Lancashire, BB9 7JS. Tel: 0800 161 3823/01282 716839; e-mail: admin@nrhp.co.uk; website: www.nrhp.co.uk.

Hypnotherapeutic approaches to working with children

12

Kathy Stephenson

CHAPTER OUTLINE

This chapter explores the issues of using hypnotherapy techniques with children. It offers a flexible practice model while highlighting a variety of approaches which harness the child's imagination. Ethical issues are addressed, along with consideration of the parent's involvement. It goes on to explore common problems, including enuresis, pain, anxiety and low self-esteem. Hypnotherapy techniques are presented through the use of case studies.

KEY WORDS

Children
Ethics
Parents
Imagery
Metaphor
Children's problems

© 2010 Elsevier Ltd.
DOI: 10.1016/B978-0-7020-3082-6.00014-9

INTRODUCTION

Working hypnotherapeutically with children can be a richly rewarding experience. It offers the opportunity to help the child utilize their own capacity to make beneficial changes and to tap into their limitless creative ability. The underpinning philosophy within this chapter is a belief that each individual child has, within themselves, all the resources they need. It offers suggestions for both therapists and child care practitioners to adopt a child-centred, flexible, responsive approach, whereby the therapist/clinician uses whatever the child brings to the therapeutic encounter to enable the child to achieve their goals.

The term 'practitioner' will be used throughout this chapter to be inclusive of both therapists (psychologists, counsellors, etc.) and clinicians (doctors, nurses, etc.). As Sugarman (2007) points out, hypnotherapy is a skill-set and strategy that bridges both physiological and psychological in both intent and outcome.

Research into hypnosis with children suggests that they are generally very good subjects for hypnotherapeutic intervention. It also suggests that they are often more hypnotically responsive than adults. They respond well to creative visualization, metaphor and pretending. In general, children have active imaginations and come along to sessions without many of the preconceived notions about hypnosis. They also tend not to analyse themselves or the process to the extent that adults do. Hilliard (1979) suggests that most of the variables suggestive of hypnotic responsiveness in adults have their precursors in the creative, affective and play experience of childhood.

There are several distinctions between working with children and adults. While adults commonly close their eyes during hypnosis, children, particularly those under the age of 10, seldom do. They often associate instructions for eye closure with being told to go to sleep and may equate it to loss of control. They are curious and do not want to miss anything. This can be somewhat disconcerting for therapists who often regard eye closure as validation of the trance experience and a sign of intensity of the hypnotic experience. This can be initially uncomfortable for the practitioner, as it moves them out of their comfort zone of eye closure and requires modification of their usual practice. Children also have a tendency to fidget and move around more than adults in hypnosis and this can be misinterpreted as a sign that the child is not in trance. Children generally learn hypnosis more easily than adults because they are frequently in and out of altered states of awareness as part of their normal development (Kohen 1990).

There is a well-documented link between hypnotic ability and stages of child development. Children aged between 4 and 6 years tend to be more responsive to a kind of 'protohypnosis' which is an absorption in fantasy games related to the external world rather than detached internal fantasy. Between the ages of 7–14 hypnotic ability is thought to be at its peak and decreases during adolescence (Hilliard & Morgan 1978). However, it is important to note that individual children vary greatly in their speed of development. Success in working with children requires the practitioner to be aware of development issues and therefore to adapt inductions and suggestions to not only the age of the child but also to be consistent with the individual child's level of intelligence, understanding of language and their cognitive and perceptual skills.

CREATIVE FLEXIBILITY

There has been a general shift over the past few decades from the authoritarian, direct approach in the field of hypnotherapy to more indirect permissive approaches pioneered by the work of psychiatrist Dr Milton Erickson. He developed an indirect style of induction, characterized by words such as 'allow yourself' and 'imagine, if you will', using ambiguous and cooperative, rather than directional language, to guide the unconscious mind into trance. Erickson used a non-directive approach, using stories and metaphors in order to distract the conscious mind, making indirect suggestions to the unconscious mind. He believed that the unconscious responds to metaphor, symbols, images and artfully vague language. His work influenced many practitioners in the field, including Dr Karen Olness, Professor of Paediatrics (foremost authority on the application of hypnosis with children). She is the co-author of the classic text: *Hypnosis and Hypnotherapy with Children* (Olness & Kohen 1996). The recipe for a successful hypnotherapeutic intervention with children, according to Olness, is using induction techniques which are permissive in nature, emphasizing the child's involvement and control and encouraging their active participation in the process of experiencing and utilizing the hypnotic state.

Hypnotherapy training courses commonly teach hypnotherapeutic techniques as a series of ordered steps: introduction, induction, deepener, therapeutic suggestion, reorientation, ratification and reflection. This process has been likened to a 'vessel' approach to hypnosis, whereby the subject is dipped into a vessel full of hypnotic trance and some subconscious change occurs during immersion. The subject then floats back to the surface, is removed from the vessel and wiped down (Teleska & Roffman 2004). This vessel approach is a useful protocol to use with adults, but less useful with children, as successful hypnotherapeutic intervention with children relies on the practitioner being creative, flexible and going with the flow. Children often arrive for consultation in their own everyday trances, drifting between fantasy and reality. This provides the opportunity to tap into their natural state of being. It can be highly effective to go with the flow of their fertile imaginations and allow the child's tenacious and self-protected autonomy to dictate the order and flow of the therapeutic outcome (Sugarman 2007).

ETHICAL CONSIDERATIONS

Working with children requires care and consideration, as children are still in the process of developing their own construction of reality. Fordyce (1988) suggests that two questions should be at the forefront of the therapist's mind when working with children. First, 'What am I teaching my client by what I say and do?' Second, 'What is my client learning?' These questions arise from the need to maintain a self-supervisory capacity and reflect sensitivity to the ongoing process of the therapeutic session.

Working with children requires the practitioner to have either formal training in paediatrics, child psychology or have taken sufficient postgraduate training and supervision with children in their respective discipline and area of expertise before using hypnosis. It also assumes appropriate training and certification in the use of hypnosis in general and its application to children (Wall 2007).

The practitioner working with children must stay within their own professional remit and know when to refer on to another appropriate professional (see Ch. 3). Children, who present with problems such as pain or enuresis, should always, without exception, be medically evaluated before commencing with hypnotherapy sessions. This is also applicable when dealing with issues such as psychological trauma, whereby the child should be referred for assessment of a child psychologist.

Contraindications to using hypnosis with children are: risking physical endangerment, risking aggravation of emotional problems, hypnosis for entertainment outside the therapeutic relationship and when more effective treatment is available (Olness & Kohen 1996).

PARENTAL INVOLVEMENT

A consideration when working with children is having parents as a contributing factor. The role of parents is significant in the overall process. Their words and actions can support or undermine the hypnotherapeutic work. The child's problem may even be due to the parent's behaviour or exacerbated by them. Kohen et al (1984) in a study of over 500 hypnotherapy sessions with children found that negative outcomes were correlated to parental over-involvement. Autonomy is required for children to effectively develop self-mastery techniques and parents 'nagging' appeared to negate the autonomy necessary for the child to take ownership of their own self-hypnosis.

The role of the parent is central to the work the practitioner does with the child. From the onset, the practitioner is dealing not only with the child but also with the parent, therefore it is vital to establish rapport with both the child and the parent. There is a fine balancing act between keeping the parents feeling they are part of the process, while also respecting the child's right to be able to speak to the practitioner about their concerns in confidence. It is important to establish open challenges of communication with parents from the beginning to ensure all concerned are working towards a common goal.

Although there are numerous benefits to using hypnotherapeutic approaches with children, there can be reluctance on the part of some parents to seek out hypnotherapy due to widespread misconceptions about hypnosis. This often comes from the perceived connotations relating to lack of control associated with stage hypnotism. This fear can be allayed by spending time to explore the myths with the parents and offer them reassurances that hypnosis is a very safe and effective therapy and the client is always in control. They may even wish to experience hypnosis themselves so they can feel comfortable with the process.

As the initial point of contact comes from the parent, this provides an opportunity for basic information gathering such as the nature of the problem, family dynamics, child's health history, etc. This initial discussion also gives the practitioner the opportunity to establish the ground rules in terms of how the therapy sessions will be conducted. In practice, the author finds it useful to conduct this initial consultation with the parent via the telephone or in person prior to meeting the child. This allows for the initial contact with the child to focus upon directly addressing them individually; giving the child the opportunity to express their perception of what is happening to them. It also gives the practitioner the opportunity to establish the child's level of motivation to change.

The initial consultation with the child enables the practitioner to gather information about the child's interests, hobbies and experiences. This information can be used later in the hypnotherapeutic process. The language used when addressing the child should be pitched at their level and should avoid being too simple, and therefore patronising, or too complex for the child to understand. The practitioner can enhance rapport by taking into account the child's perceptual and conceptual skills with regard to both the problem and the possible solutions.

It is important within any initial hypnotherapy session with either an adult or a child, that they can define or perceive a desired therapeutic outcome. While working with children, it is useful to remember that the desired outcome of the parent or indeed the practitioner may be different from the desired outcome of the child. This can be addressed by directly asking the child: 'Am I right in understanding that what you want is ...?' (e.g. to stop biting your nails). Alternatively, the practitioner can set up an ideomotor response during the hypnotic induction and after asking a series of general yes/no questions, can pose the question about the desired outcome.

The solution-focused 'miracle' question can be beneficial in ensuring that the child is engaged in the process and it also enables them to see beyond their condition and set positive outcomes for the future. This helps to give them motivation to change and this is an important variable in the success of the hypnotherapeutic intervention. For example:

> *Imagine if when you go home today and later you go to bed and go to sleep as usual, during the night a miracle happens and makes the (problem) disappear. Now, because you were asleep, you don't know anything about this so it is quite a surprise for you .... So, this miracle has happened. What's going to be the first thing that surprises you today and lets you know that something amazing happened last night? What else? What would your family and friends see you doing that would tell them something amazing had happened? What else will have changed?*

The feedback can later be woven into any future orientation suggestions in hypnosis using the language the child uses. Also the absence of symptoms can be translated into beginnings of new future behaviours (Berg 2003).

The child will benefit from the knowledge that hypnosis is not something done to them. It is something that the child does for themselves. As the child progresses throughout the sessions, it is useful to focus on the fact that they

Hypnotherapeutic approaches to working with children

have made the changes themselves. Therefore the symptoms do not just go away; something the child did made it better. So for example if the child who bites his/her nails does not do this for a few days the practitioner may say, 'I wonder what you did to make it better.' A central theme of the hypnotherapeutic inductions and suggestions is the focus on the child's own involvement and control in the overall process. Directing questions to the child allows them to answer directly for themselves. If the parent persistently answers for the child, refocus on the child by saying, 'OK so that is how your Mum would answer my question and what do you think?'

Children are not always as forthcoming as adults when describing their conditions and often need gentle prompting such as 'What can you tell me about xxx?'; 'How does having xxx make you feel?'; 'Is this a problem for anyone else?' Once the practitioner has elicited the symptoms in the child's own words, it is useful to use these words when feeding back to the child. This helps to establish rapport and allows the child to feel understood.

ESTABLISHING RAPPORT

Rapport is an essential baseline for effective communication. It helps the practitioner to communicate at a deep level with the child and to gain their trust.

When the practitioner establishes rapport and paces the child's experience, they can then lead the child towards the direction appropriate to meet their outcome. The role of the practitioner is to be a guide for the child, helping them to use their imagination rather than imposing changes. They can lead them towards a better state or towards some new ideas. Leading assumes a positive intention and enables the practitioner to subtly take the child in a new direction.

When introducing the child to hypnosis, it is helpful to tell them that it is very similar to daydreaming, pretending or imagining. It is therefore something they already know how to do but maybe they did not know that they knew they could use this to help themselves to solve the problem they are experiencing.

HARNESSING THE POWER OF THE CHILD'S IMAGINATION

Children have the most wonderful imaginations. They drift easily between fantasy and reality and therefore it is relatively easy for most children to achieve an altered state of consciousness. This is a very familiar and comfortable state common to their experience and it is therefore very easy to harness and utilize the vivid power of a child's imagination. As children play, they use their imaginations in many ways. They are experts in fantasy and skilled at pretending and make-believe. The key to successful hypnotherapeutic intervention with children is to harness the power of their rich and fertile creative imaginations, to go with the flow and utilize what they bring to the therapy session.

One highly effective hypnotherapeutic tool to use with children to harness the power of their imagination is the metaphorical approach. Throughout history, metaphorical stories such as *Aesop's Fables* and *Homer's Tales*, have been used to convey messages, and reinforce moral and societal values. Metaphors convey messages in indirect ways using symbolic language. A practitioner can deliver a message directly to the unconscious mind, bypassing the critical barriers of the conscious mind. Metaphors in hypnotherapy are designed as a form of indirect, imaginative and implied communication with the child about experiences and outcomes that may help to find resolutions. What disguises therapeutic metaphors from other types of stories or anecdotes is that they are purposely designed symbolic communication with specific therapeutic intention (Burns 2005).

Metaphors enable the practitioner to communicate with both the conscious and unconscious simultaneously. Therefore as the conscious mind listens to the symbolic rich story and processes the words, the therapeutic message goes into the unconscious mind and searches for meanings, personalized relevance and resolutions. Research into the therapeutic use of metaphor with children by Crowley and Mills (1986) suggests that the use of metaphor is a successful communication tool that appears to mediate therapeutic change in a pleasant and imaginative way. Metaphors allow the child to be exposed to different perspectives and explore new possibilities to allow them to create their own changes. This is also a very gentle non-threatening way for children to view and re-frame the problems they are experiencing. Kuttner (1998) found that hypnotherapeutic intervention involving storytelling and imagery was significantly more effective than behavioural techniques or standard medical practice in alleviating distress during bone marrow procedures in young children with leukaemia. Stories with positive suggestions and entwined and embedded commands enable children to make beneficial changes and develop new innovative ways to overcome limitations, while viewing the problem as something that is happening to someone else.

SPECIFIC CONDITIONS

Hypnotherapy has been used as an effective tool to help children overcome a wide range of conditions. It has been used to overcome phobias (Hatzenbuehler & Schroder 1978), in the control of pain (Olness & Kohen 1996), with sleep disturbances and nightmares (King et al 1989). It has also been used successfully in paediatric oncology to alleviate chemotherapy-related nausea and vomiting (Hawkins et al 1995).

There are many techniques which can be employed when working with children, notably dissociation, re-framing, anchoring, suggestion, creative visualization and metaphors. A practical application of these techniques and case study examples will be explored in the following section. The intention is to illustrate examples of interactive co-creative processes, as opposed to prescriptive imagery and scripts.

ENURESIS

The most common childhood condition which I deal with in my practice is nocturnal enuresis or bed wetting (Box 12.1). Under the age of 6 years old, enuresis should be considered a normal development variant. Children

BOX 12.1 Case study 1

Jonathan was 8 years old when he came to see me. He had just started the Cubs (junior part of the Scouts movement) and a camping trip had been planned, which was causing both Jonathan and his Mother much anxiety. He had occasionally wet his bed since he was young, but the frequency had increased over the last few months when friends had started to have 'sleep overs'. He had avoided the overnight stays with friends and what had been a peripheral issue had become a central concern. The more anxious he became, the more he experienced enuresis. During the first session, we discussed how the body works. Mindful of the age of the child, we used simple drawings of the brain, bladder and urethra and also drew a toilet and a tap. We put the tap on the bladder which was full of 'wee, wee' (Jonathan's word for urine). As Jonathan enjoyed playing on his home computer, we imagined his brain as a big computer. The computer sends massages to all parts of the body. I asked him if he could send a message from the computer brain to his legs to make them move about and his head to nod and so on. I then asked him to send a message to his eyes to close and all of his body to relax. This was a simple yet very effective induction and soon, Jonathan was in the control room in his brain. I asked if he could check out if the link between his computer and the part that controls his legs was working properly, he nodded. We spent the next few minutes checking other 'links' until eventually, I asked him to examine the link between the computer brain and his bladder tap. He said it sometimes worked but other times didn't. So I asked him to spend some time fixing the problem. After several minutes of silence, he opened his eyes wide and said he had installed a new computer link! His Mother rang several weeks later to say he had remained dry at night and enjoyed Cub camp. Jonathan had managed to take ownership of his problem, developed an understanding of how his body and mind worked together and used the power of his imagination to take back control in a resourceful way.

who present with this problem over the age of 6 years should have possible physical causes such as urinary tract problems ruled out via medical examination. Bed wetting can have significant negative social implications.

MEDICAL PROCEDURES

An effective technique to use with children undergoing medical procedures is the trance phenomenon disassociation, whereby the child experiences their body, mind or feelings as separate from themselves. This enables the child to put a barrier or some distance between themselves and any discomfort. This technique is very useful in dental treatment, for example, suggesting to the child that they can imagine going to their own special place (Box 12.2). The child is asked to imagine a place where they would feel safe and comfortable; this can perhaps be a place familiar to them or created in their imagination.

Dissociation is a very useful tool to use to help a child feel more comfortable and in control when undergoing a variety of medical procedures such as lumbar punctures, bone marrow biopsies and chemotherapy. Liossi's (1999) review of a range of research studies indicted the usefulness of hypnosis as an effective intervention for the control of pain and anxiety associated with medical procedures.

BOX 12.2 Case study 2

Jilly aged 9 came to see me due to her increasing anxiety about ongoing dental treatment. After exploring her interests, hobbies, likes and dislikes, Jilly established a special place on a beautiful multi-coloured flying carpet. She imagined flying high into the sky on her safe and special magic carpet, landing in wonderful lands and experiencing exciting adventures. She practiced visualizing climbing on to the dentist chair as climbing onto her magic carpet and soon began to re-frame the experience of visiting the dentist as an opportunity to experience a wonderful adventure. She reported feeling a sense of control when she had previously experienced a sense of helplessness. During each visit to the dentist she remained calm and entranced throughout the whole procedure.

The use of hypnosis with children undergoing medical procedures has many advantages. It is safe and does not produce unpleasant side-effects. There is no reduction of mental capacity and no development of tolerance to the hypnotic effect. It can help the child to develop a sense of control and personal sense of mastery.

REDUCING ANXIETY AND BUILDING SELF-ESTEEM

Hypnotherapeutic suggestions can help to build self-esteem and reduce anxiety (Box 12.3). Children can often get caught up in a cycle of worry about a whole variety of things from concern about friendship groups, anxiety about performing well at school and adapting to changes at home. Just in the same way as adults often do, children can make themselves quite anxious about many things and this can lead to developing some of the physical symptoms of stress such as upset digestion, insomnia and lack of concentration. Hypnosis can help children to break the cycle of worry and learn to accept that sometimes life is a challenge, and that they are more than capable to rise above any challenges and deal with things in a calm and positive manner. Children are often very receptive to learning new ways to regain a sense of control. Relaxation techniques, role play and creative imagery can help them to feel empowered. Cognitive-behavioural approaches and positive hypnotherapeutic suggestions can help the child to feel good within themselves and about themselves, increase their levels of self-confidence and bring about a calmness of mind. It can also help them to be free of anxious stressful thoughts.

MANAGING PAIN

Hypnosis is an effective method for controlling pain. This approach is based on the premise that the processes of the mind have a direct effect on the body. At the mind/brain level, many children are able to distort their own perception, so that they experience deep levels of anaesthesia using hypnosis. At brain/body level, increased endorphins, the body's own natural pain killer, have been recorded in clients following hypnotherapy sessions (Rossi & Cheek 1988).

BOX 12.3 Case study 3

David, aged 10, came along to see me with his father. He had recently moved from another part of the country and was feeling very anxious and reluctant to go to school. He had attended the new school for 2 months and initially seemed to be accepted into the group of young boys who played football during lunch time. After a few weeks, things began to change. Several boys began to laugh at David's clothes, accent and mannerisms. He experienced name-calling and cheering taunts and began to avoid the playground whenever possible. David was very upset and found it difficult to concentrate on his school work. I spent some time finding out about David's hobbies and favourite programmes. He enjoyed football and watching Spiderman, the movie. During the session, I asked David what he thought Spiderman would be like if he was to encounter the bullies on the playground. David sat quietly for several minutes with his eyes opened staring at the wall; after a little while he looked at me and nodded. It transpired that he was watching Spiderman on the movie on the wall in my office. I asked if he would like to watch it again and talk me through it. As Spiderman dealt with the bullies in a calm and confident way, I asked David to step into the movie and to notice what it feels like to respond to the bullies in this way. We used a confidence anchor and then ran the movie through again with David being himself and responding to the bullying in the same calm and confident way. In addition to this I used ego strengthening suggestions to reinforce the positive scenario. There was no formal induction, deepener or hypnosis script used, just the imagery David presented, which was used to draw upon his own inner resources. During the next session, David learnt how to use self-hypnosis. Within 2 weeks of the first session, his parents rang to say David was back to his normal self, had settled at school and the bullying had ceased.

The history of hypnosis demonstrates the use of pain management from the amputations of surgeon James Esdaile through to the current use of hypno-sedation. There are numerous clinic research studies on the use of hypnosis in pain management (Olness 1987, Kuttner 1988).

It is important to remember that pain is in a sense a warning signal and therefore the practitioner must ensure that the child's parent has sought medical advice before doing pain management work.

Children tend to respond very well to making changes to the size, shape, colour and temperature of their pain. While taking the case history, it is useful to ask the child to describe the sensory modalities of pain, e.g. the kinesthetic sensations of the pain such as sharp, pounding, heavy, dull, twisting, tingling, stabbing, etc. They may also describe thermal sensations such as hot, boiling or cold. As the child describes their pain, it is useful to take note of the metaphorical references, e.g. 'The pain is like a hammer pounding away in my head.' You can ask them to close their eyes and imagine what the pain looks like and to describe the imagery of pain such as shape, texture, size, colour and even sound. This information gathering serves two useful purposes. First, it helps the child to feel understood and therefore enhances rapport. Second, it gives you information to work with in hypnosis.

Hypnotherapy can also help to alter the child's perception of pain by helping to alter the interpretation they put on pain. You can suggest in hypnosis that the child can substitute the painful sensation for a less unpleasant sensation such as a tingle or an itch. This is particularly useful for clients who need to continue to be aware of the stimulus of the pain. For example:

You can be surprised and delighted to find that the stabbing hot sensation becomes a cool gentle tingling and you can notice that cool gentle tingling now ... that's right ...

Displacement of the locus of pain is another very useful method of pain control using hypnosis. The pain can be displaced to another area of the body to a less vulnerable less painful area from the ear to the toe, for example. The practitioner can also continue this and suggest the client moves it outside the body. One poignant example of this type of pain control is the case of my own daughter (Box 12.4).

BOX 12.4 Case study 4

At the age of 12, Jess developed migraines. Although tablets helped ease the pain she would feel nauseous and completely wiped out for hours and had to lie down in a darkened room. The migraines occurred once or twice a month over a 12-month period and her GP said the migraines could be hormone-related and she would eventually grow out of them. One day I was out shopping with Jess and she developed a migraine. I brought her home and before giving her the usual medication, I asked if she would like to try some hypnotherapy. She had experienced and enjoyed some general relaxation techniques previously and agreed to give it a go. She lay down on her bed and closed her eyes and I did a general induction and then modality change work. She imagined the pain she was experiencing as a large bright red throbbing blob which covered the whole of her forehead. We worked through a process of making changes to each modality. She imagined slightly shrinking the blob and making it throb a little less. Then she softened the edges and twirled and swirled it around until it turned into a very small red ball. I suggested she might like to try to change the colour of the ball and she changed it to a pale pink colour. After a few minutes the ball stopped moving and shrunk down even further to a small pinkish dot in the centre of her forehead. I asked her what she would like to do with this now; some children suggest turning it to mist and letting it evaporate, others dissolve it or simply blow it away. Jess said she would like to give it to me but didn't want me to feel hurt. I promptly replied that it would not hurt me as I would throw it straight out of the window. She decided to imagine it leaving her forehead and floating out of the window and away. We ended the session and I left her to rest. Within 10 minutes she was pain free and out playing happily in the garden. From that day on she controlled her migraines herself whether at school or at home; she simply used the power of her imagination. She adapted this in other innovative ways. When a dry cough was preventing her from concentrating at school, she imaged the cough as a fierce tiger. She then soothingly stroked the tiger and it turned into a little kitten in her imagination and this helped the cough to calm down. Within 6 months she had grown out of the migraines and as she grew older she also stopped using the self-hypnosis techniques. As a 17-year-old, this is a common response, I just hope she will return to harness the power of her imagination in adulthood.

Hypnotherapeutic approaches to working with children

THE GIFT OF SELF-HYPNOSIS

A wonderful gift to give to children during the therapy sessions is to teach them self-hypnosis. This enables them to actively participate in the treatment process and to reinforce self-mastery. Karen Olness's (Olness & Kohen 1996) research into school children using self-hypnosis to change immune response, including both humoral and cellular response suggests that all children with chronic conditions such as haemophilia, cancer, diabetes and sickle cell disease should have the opportunity to learn self-hypnosis as soon as possible after the diagnosis is established.

Australian paediatrician, Dr Hewson-Bower's research into hypnotherapeutic intervention demonstrated that children who learnt to practice self-hypnosis have reduced numbers of respiratory infections and fewer days' illness when they do contract a respiratory infection (Hewson-Bower & Drummond 1996). Hawkins and Polemikos (2002) found that school-aged children who were experiencing sleep disturbances following a trauma benefited from learning self-hypnosis. In a controlled trial conducted by Olness (1987), self-hypnosis was shown to be significantly more effective than either pain killers or placebo in reducing the frequency of migraine headaches in children between the ages of 6 and 12 years of age. Teaching children self-hypnosis helps them to cope with stressful and challenging events using these self-mastery techniques as transferable skills. Evidence suggests that many young people continue to transfer the skills learnt in one context to other challenges and to learn for example, to control habits, prevent migraine and control anxiety (Kohen et al 1984).

SUMMARY

Working hypnotherapeutically with children requires a responsive adaptable approach on the part of the practitioner. It allows the practitioner to be inventive, playful and spontaneous and to build a strong therapeutic relationship with the child while providing symptom relief (Liossi 1999). When working with children using hypnotherapeutic techniques, it is useful to remember that hypnosis with children is easy but not simple, it is fun but requires concentration and it should be conducted with respect for the child and their intrinsic abilities (Kohen 1990). Successful intervention is based on harnessing the power of the child's rich imagination and working with the child in a flexible, creative and responsive way. If practitioners wish to successfully work with a child, then they must modify the inductions and suggestions so they are compatible with the age of the child. The case study examples offered all have a common theme of working without set scripts in a spontaneous way, taking what the child offers and incorporating it into various well-known techniques such as disassociation, anchoring and creative visualization. The techniques all involved pacing the child's experience and leading the child into a more resourceful state to achieve a successful outcome.

REFERENCES

Berg, I., 2003. Children's solution work. Norton, London.

Burns, G., 2005. 101 Healing stories for kids and teens. John Wiley, London.

Crowley, R., Mills, J., 1986. Therapeutic metaphors for children. Routledge, London.

Fordyce, W.E., 1988. Pain and suffering. Am. Psychol. 43, 276–283.

Hatzenbuehler, L., Schroder, H., 1978. Desensitisation procedures in the treatment of childhood disorders. Psychol. Bull. 85, 831–844.

Hawkins, P., Polemikos, N., 2002. Hypnosis treatment of sleeping problems in children experiencing loss. Contemporary Hypnosis 19 (1), 18–24.

Hawkins, P., Liossi, C., Ewart, B., et al., 1995. Hypnotherapy for control of anticipatory nausea and vomiting in children with cancer: preliminary findings. Psychooncology 4, 101–106.

Hewson-Bower, B., Drummond, P.D., 1996. Secretory immunoglobulin A increases during relaxation in children with and without recurring upper respiratory tract infections. J. Dev. Behav. Pediatr. 17 (5), 311–316.

Hilliard, J., 1979. Personality and hypnosis. Chicago Press, Chicago.

Hilliard, J., Morgan, A., 1978. Treatment of anxiety and pain in childhood cancer through hypnosis. In: Frankel, H. (Ed.), Hypnosis. New York Press, New York.

King, N., Cranstoun, F., Josephs, A., 1989. Emotive imagery and children's nighttimes fears. J. Behav. Ther. Exp. Psychiatry 20 (20), 125–135.

Kohen, D., 1990. A hypnotherapeutic approach to enuresis. In: Hammond, D. (Ed.), Handbook of hypnotic suggestions and metaphors. Norton, London.

Kohen, D., Coldwell, S., Heimel, A., 1984. The use of relaxation/mental imagery in Tourette Syndrome. Am. J. Clin. Hypn. 29 (4), 227–237.

Kuttner, L., 1988. Favorite stories: a hypnotic pain-reduction technique for children in acute pain. Am. J. Clin. Hypn. 30, 289–295.

Kuttner, L., 1998. No fears no tears 13 years on – video tape. Fanlight Productions, New York.

Liossi, C., 1999. Management of paediatric procedure-related cancer pain. Pain Reviews 6, 279–302.

Olness, K., 1987. Headaches in children. Paediatrics in Review 8, 307–311.

Olness, K., Kohen, D., 1996. Hypnosis and hypnotherapy with children. Guilford Press, New York.

Rossi, E., Cheek, D., 1988. Mind body therapy. Norton, London.

Sugarman, L., 2007. Hypnosis with children: a contextual framework. In: Wester, W., Sugarman, L. (Eds.), Therapeutic hypnosis with children and adolescents. Crown House, Carmarthen.

Teleska, J., Roffman, A., 2004. A continuum of hypnotherapeutic interactions: from formal hypnosis to hypnotic conversation. American Society of Clinical Hypnosis 47, 103–116.

Wall, T.W., 2007. Ethical considerations with children and hypnosis. In: Wester, W., Sugarman, L. (Eds.), Therapeutic hypnosis with children and adolescents. Crown House, Carmarthen.

FURTHER READING

Wester, W., Sugarman, L., 2007. Therapeutic hypnosis with children and adolescents. Crown House, Carmarthen.

USEFUL RESOURCES

Hypnotherapy Training and Practitioners – www.general-hypnotherapy-register.com.

Self-hypnosis: audio CDs and weekend workshops –www.innerchange.co.uk.

13 Hypno-psychotherapy for functional gastrointestinal disorders

Elizabeth Taylor

CHAPTER OUTLINE

Impaired quality of life and emotional distress are common in functional gastrointestinal disorders. Although well-established diagnostic criteria exist, many patients undergo exhaustive medical investigations. Repeated negative procedures increase both patient anxiety and healthcare costs. There is growing awareness that these disorders result from biological, environmental and psychosocial factors, with published evidence supporting the clinical efficacy of various combinations of psychological therapies. More extensive physician training is required if these disorders are to be assessed and treated effectively.

KEY WORDS

Gastrointestinal disorders
IBS
CBT
Gut-directed hypnotherapy

© 2010 Elsevier Ltd.
DOI: 10.1016/B978-0-7020-3082-6.00015-0

Functional gastrointestinal disorders (FGID) are conditions in which people complain of symptoms for which no organic cause can be found. They affect up to 20% of western populations (Sandler 1990, Drossman et al 1993) with recent evidence suggesting they are equally common in the Third World (Spiller 2005). Although FGID are frequently presented in primary care and account for approximately half of the gastroenterologists' workload (Thompson 2006), they are considered challenging by many doctors. This is not surprising as FGID is characterized by multiple recurring physical symptoms in the absence of known structural or biochemical cause. Additionally, sufferers have a higher prevalence of emotional problems and traumatic life events than healthy subjects or patients with organic disease (Creed 1999, Douglas & Drossman 1999). Time restrictions, together with lack of training or motivation to elicit psychosocial concerns have caused frustration, misunderstanding and compromised doctor–patient relationships (Toner et al 1998). Diagnostic pathways have added to the problem. FGID were traditionally diagnosed by excluding organic pathology which resulted in multiple consultations, excessive investigations, over-prescribing and a disproportionate utilization of healthcare resources (Jones et al 2007). Describing functional disorders by what they are not rather than what they are, e.g. 'we can't find anything wrong with you!' suggests that the doctor does not believe the patient when he/she complains of physical symptoms and impaired quality of life. The difficulty in establishing a positive diagnosis and poor response to conventional treatment serve to erode the patient's confidence in the medical profession (Talley et al 1995).

Over the last three decades, this unsatisfactory situation has been addressed by the formulation and development of the Rome criteria (Thompson 2006). Specialist teams meet in Rome to develop and update positive diagnostic criteria and treatment recommendations for FGID. The latter can be reliably diagnosed using these criteria providing there are no 'alarm' features indicative of organic disease (Spiller 2005).

This chapter will focus on irritable bowel syndrome (IBS) and functional dyspepsia as they are the most commonly reported FGID (Box 13.1). However, at REAL Wellbeing (a charitable organization situated in Northern England), patients with functional dyspepsia and other functional GI disorders usually present with a diagnosis of IBS with reference to upper GI tract problems and predominant bowel habit (diarrhoea or constipation predominant). For the purpose of this chapter, it can be assumed that IBS is a blanket term for FGID with treatment adapted to individual need. The symptomatology of IBS will be described, followed by a brief explanation of the therapeutic content of dynamic psychotherapy, cognitive-behaviour therapy and gut-directed hypnotherapy. Selected research demonstrating the efficacy of these approaches is outlined together with suggested reasons for their effectiveness in IBS. The main focus of the chapter will be a national study which assessed the feasibility of the provision of group therapy in routine care using a standardized treatment protocol (Taylor et al 2004a). Congruent with most studies, the latter is reported

> **BOX 13.1 Classification of functional gastrointestinal and bowel disorders (excerpts from the Rome II criteria)**
>
> **I. Gastrointestinal disorders**
> A. Functional dyspepsia
> B. Dysmotility-like dyspepsia
> C. Unspecified (non-specific) dyspepsia
>
> **II. Bowel disorders**
> A. Irritable bowel syndrome (IBS)
> B. Functional abdominal bloating
> C. Functional constipation
> D. Functional diarrhoea
> E. Unspecified functional bowel disorder
>
> Diagnostic criteria for IBS
> At least 12 weeks, which need not be consecutive, in the preceding 12 months, of abdominal discomfort or pain that has two or three features:
> 1. Pain relieved with defecation; and/or
> 2. Onset associated with a change in frequency or stool; and/or
> 3. Onset associated with a change in form (appearance) of stool.
>
> Diagnostic criteria for functional dyspepsia
> At least 12 weeks, which need not be consecutive, in the preceding 12 months, of:
> 1. Persistent or recurrent dyspepsia (pain or discomfort centred in the upper abdomen); and
> 2. No evidence of organic disease (including at upper endoscopy) that is likely to explain the symptoms; and
> 3. No evidence that dyspepsia is exclusively relieved by defecation or associated with the onset of a change in stool frequency or stool form, i.e. not IBS.
> The classification scheme for functional gastrointestinal and bowel disorders (FGID) is shown. Diagnostic criteria for IBS and functional dyspepsia, the two most common FGID are also listed.
>
> (Cited in Jones et al 2007.)

from the quantitative perspective, so in order to establish which elements of the programme were the most effective and valued the greatest by participants, a post-intervention qualitative evaluation will be discussed. As treatment-seeking IBS patients are predominantly female, this study additionally allows the experiences of male sufferers to be expressed. The therapists' views are also presented. The chapter will conclude with recommendations for education, training and development.

DEFINITION, SYMPTOMS AND TREATMENTS

IBS describes a collection of symptoms causing muscle spasm and irritation in the lower gastrointestinal tract. The three central symptoms of IBS are abdominal pain, bloating and disordered bowel habit (classical IBS). Atypical IBS refers to patients with just one or two of the central symptoms

(Whorwell 1987). Many additional gastrointestinal (GI) symptoms are reported such as early satiety, nausea, vomiting, indigestion, heartburn, gastro-oesophageal reflux, anal pain and incomplete evacuation. Patients also report a wide range of non-gastrointestinal symptoms, including headaches, lethargy, musculoskeletal, gynaecological and urological problems. Standard medical intervention is targeted towards symptom reduction, including antispasmodic, diarrhoeal/laxative, acid suppressant, antidepressant medication, etc. Some patients respond to exclusion diets and others to probiotics. There is increasing evidence, however, suggesting the pathophysiology of IBS is multifactorial, with environmental issues, gender, visceral sensitivity, gut flora alterations and psychosocial stressors all playing a part. Symptoms are thought to be associated with altered 5-HT transmission and central processing of noxious stimuli (Jones et al 2007, Clark & DeLegge 2008). Treatment can only be effective if the complex relationship between these factors is acknowledged and addressed. Assessment and treatment, therefore, needs to integrate gut function with psychosocial issues (Levy et al 2006). Research into dynamic psychotherapy, CBT and hypnotherapy has provided ample evidence of efficacy in IBS.

DYNAMIC PSYCHOTHERAPY

Dynamic psychotherapy owes much to Freud's identification of the unconscious mind and ego defence mechanisms such as repression. Rarely complete, repression manifests itself into psychological symptoms or psychosomatic disorder. Although modern, brief focussed methodology is used; today, the aim is the same, i.e. to facilitate self-understanding by means of therapeutic regression, enabling the patient to relinquish the defence and adopt more adaptive behaviours.

In an early randomized controlled trial, Guthrie et al (1991) found that patients who had received exploratory dynamic psychotherapy demonstrated a superior reduction in IBS symptoms, improved quality of life and reduction in healthcare costs compared with usual medical treatment. This finding was supported in a more recent study. Creed et al (2003) randomly assigned patients with severe IBS to one of three conditions, i.e. eight sessions of individual dynamic psychotherapy; 20 mg daily of antidepressant medication (paroxetine), or standard medical care. Three months after the intervention, outcome measures (SF-36) demonstrated superior improvements in the physical aspects of health-related quality of life in both psychotherapy and paroxetine conditions compared with treatment as usual. At the 12-month follow-up, psychotherapy only was associated with significantly reduced healthcare costs compared with standard medical care.

COGNITIVE BEHAVIOUR THERAPY

Cognitive behaviour therapy (CBT) describes clinical problems as disorders of thought and feelings. As behaviour is controlled by thought, the most effective way to change maladaptive behaviour is to change the underlying

Hypno-psychotherapy for functional gastrointestinal disorders

maladaptive thinking (Beck 1993). The relationships between thoughts, feelings, behaviours and GI symptoms are explored, using techniques of cognitive restructuring to produce lasting change. CBT combines techniques such as cognitive approaches with stress management, pain management, assertiveness training and relaxation to provide a multi-component intervention (Toner 2005).

Trials of cognitive therapy have shown symptomatic and psychological improvement, compared with a similar period of daily symptom monitoring (Greene & Blanchard 1994). Additionally, when combined with behavioural techniques, improvements of bowel symptoms were sustained for 4 years (Neff & Blanchard 1987). In a large-scale ($n = 431$) randomized trial, Drossman et al (2003) found CBT to be more effective than attention placebo control.

When CBT was applied to groups, clinical improvements were greater than either attention placebo or standard care controls (Toner et al 1998), waiting list controls (Payne & Blanchard 1995) or support and symptom monitoring (van Dulmen et al 1996).

GUT-DIRECTED HYPNOTHERAPY

Hypnotherapy is described elsewhere in this book (see Ch. 1). Gut-directed hypnotherapy (GDHT) however, is hypnosis targeted towards the gut. In a seminal study, Whorwell et al (1984) randomly assigned 30 patients with severe refractory IBS to seven sessions of GDHT; seven sessions of supportive discussion plus placebo medication; or waiting list controls. Hypnotherapy patients demonstrated the greatest improvement in pain, bloating and bowel habit, disturbance with no relapse after 3 months. Improvement was maintained at later follow-up sessions (Whorwell et al 1987).

Further research has demonstrated economic benefits for hypnotherapy. Patients who received GDHT visited their doctors less frequently. Some returned to or obtained work, thus reducing sickness benefit claims (Houghton et al 1996, Gonsalkorale et al 2003). Reduced medication following hypnotherapy has also been reported (Koutsomanis 1997, Gonsalkorale et al 2003).

Recent studies with medium- to long-term follow-up supports the success of GDHT in adults (Gonsalkorale et al 2002, 2003, Barabasz & Barabasz 2006), and in children (Vlieger et al 2007). Group hypnotherapy is equally effective (Harvey et al 1989, Taylor et al 2004a).

WHY ARE PSYCHOLOGICAL THERAPIES BENEFICIAL IN FGID?

There is increasing evidence that IBS is a multifactorial disorder of brain–gut function. Cognitive and emotional areas of the brain modify gut motility and visceral sensitivity (Toner 2005, Clark & DeLegge 2008). Psychological distress, past traumatic experiences and recent stressors affect mood and alter gut function (Levy et al 2006). Motility abnormalities, in turn, have psychological consequences, e.g. fear of going out due to rectal urgency, fear of intimacy due to pain, food phobia, embarrassment due to wind, fear of upsetting loved ones and so on. The poor response to pharmacology, therefore, is not surprising.

Dynamic psychotherapy helps the patient to identify the relationship between past and present traumas/stressors. Similarly, CBT explores the relationship between thoughts, feelings, behaviours and GI symptoms. By adjusting cognitions and behaviour, patients are enabled to develop more adaptive ways of managing IBS and improving quality of life (Toner 2005). Cognitive change has also been demonstrated in hypnotherapy by restructuring IBS-related thoughts (Gonsalkorale et al 2004). Additionally, hypnosis has adjusted the sensory and motor component of the gastrocolonic response in IBS (Simren et al 2004) and reduced rectal sensitivity and pain sensitivity (Lea et al 2003). Palsson et al (2002), however, found rectal pain thresholds, rectal smooth muscle tone and autonomic functioning, measured before and after treatment, were unaffected by hypnotherapy. These workers argue that the latter improves IBS symptoms by reducing emotional distress and somatization. The mechanism underpinning the clinical efficacy of hypnotherapy is not yet understood but there is evidence to indicate that gastrointestinal physiology can be altered by hypnosis (Whorwell et al 1992, Whorwell 2009), similar hypotheses exist for CBT (Lackner et al 2007).

Inevitably, methodological criticism has been directed towards this literature in terms of sample size, lack of parallel comparisons with other treatments, inadequate control conditions, failure to identify primary vs secondary outcome measures, etc. (Toner 2005, Whitehead 2006, Wilson et al 2006). Nevertheless, systematic reviews to assess the quality of research into psychological treatments have indicated that these interventions are effective in reducing IBS symptoms compared with pooled controls (Lackner et al 2004). Indeed, hypnotherapy for IBS has recently been included in the NICE (2008) guidelines for primary care commissioning.

WHAT ABOUT THE PATIENT?

IBS is much misunderstood in general society and often equated with psychological disorders. Patients, especially women, often feel their embarrassing problems are trivialized and may suffer in silence for many years (Toner et al 1998, Toner 2005), adding social isolation to their difficulties. Better results may be obtained by combining hypnotherapy with CBT (Kirsch et al 1995, Schoenberger 2000) and, because of the many and diverse problems associated with IBS, a combined treatment programme would offer enhanced management. It is important for therapists and patients to work in collaboration to elicit problems and empower changes that are meaningful to the patient. CBT techniques are usually borrowed from approaches to treat anxiety and depression rather than using specific treatment protocols for IBS. Furthermore, studies reported from the quantitative framework may restrict understanding of the individual patient's and therapist's interpretation of events. As a consequence, they limit the opportunity to refine interventions more specifically to meet the needs of an individual. Only one study reported the experiences of women who received CBT for IBS (Toner et al 1998). Although treatment-seeking patients are predominantly women, little is known about men's experiences of treatment (Spiller 2005). Additionally, the results of randomized controlled trials are infrequently implemented in clinical practice (Haines & Jones 1994). Indeed, many doctors still insist on exhaustive medical investigations before they are prepared to diagnose IBS (Jones et al 2007). Moreover, facilities providing routine psychological care for this patient population are rare.

Some of these issues were addressed by ELIHC. Taylor et al (2004a) assessed the feasibility and short-term effectiveness of combined group CBT, hypnotherapy and education. The treatment protocol was standardized in a session-by-session manual and tested in a pilot group. Thereafter, 13 therapists delivered the programme to 23 different groups. A total of 158 patients (120 females, 38 males) completed group therapy.

The intervention consisted of 3-hourly sessions over a 16-week period. The initial 1.5 h consisted of CBT specific to IBS (Greene & Blanchard 1994). This focussed principally on the exploration of how certain cognitions and behaviours can influence IBS symptoms and associated psychosocial distress. Negative automatic thoughts were challenged and task-orientated assignments practised to induce greater coping abilities and the reduction of psychological and gastrointestinal symptoms. Following a short refreshment break, the educational element was delivered. This included the pathophysiology of IBS, the physiology of emotion, pain and hyperventilation, the nature of catastrophizing/perfectionistic thought, life-events, diet and the effects of multiple medical consultations and the influences of these factors on IBS. The final 20 min consisted of gut-directed hypnotherapy. After induction of hypnosis and ego-strengthening suggestions, patients were asked to place their hands on the abdomen and generate feelings of warmth and comfort in this area. This was followed by suggestions of symptom reduction and personal control over bowel function, reinforced by guided imagery (Whorwell et al 1984). Patients with upper gut problems used appropriate visualization to facilitate gastric emptying. Patients were encouraged to take responsibility for their disorder and to practise cognitive restructuring, learned coping skills and gut-directed hypnotherapy on a daily basis. Symptom and thought monitoring diaries were provided, together with standardized hypnotherapy tapes to facilitate the process. An action plan was completed at the 10th session for the purposes of self-assessment and future goal setting. During the course of the intervention, patients joined a guided walk with available public conveniences, in order to overcome incontinence phobias and encourage social interaction.

On completion of the intervention, participants completed a semi-structured qualitative questionnaire. Therapists provided detailed written reports for each session conducted. A thematic content analysis reflecting both patients' and therapists' perceptions were undertaken (Taylor et al 2004b).

Quantitative measures indicated a low attrition and high attendance rate, emphasizing the acceptance of the intervention. Outcome measures demonstrated highly significant improvements in both gastrointestinal and psychosocial symptoms. This suggests that combined psychotherapy and hypnotherapy is a feasible method for helping large numbers of patients with IBS, by providing them with advanced coping skills. Since this was a study of feasibility conducted in a lay setting, we did not include a control group. The results could therefore be susceptible to regression to the mean, though data on the natural history suggest that even with medical treatment, IBS is a chronic condition that in most patients can last for many years (Heaton & Thompson 1999).

PARTICIPANTS' VIEWS

To protect confidentiality alternative names have been used when reporting responses from participants. The primary themes identified from the patients' written responses included Accepting Help, Symptom Control and Patient Satisfaction, and Service Improvements.

ACCEPTING HELP

It is recognized that accepting help through group therapy can be anxiety-provoking. Patients frequently express concerns about sharing their personal thoughts and feelings with a group of strangers, questioning the benefits and having concerns about possible harm. Similar views were reported by the present sample, e.g.

> I didn't think that talking about problems would help. I was anxious about how I would get on with the other group members.

Several participants (15%) had pre-conceived negative beliefs about hypno-therapy with 12% expressing this as their main concern, supporting former reports of involuntary mind control (Hendler & Redd 1986), e.g.

> The hypnotherapy worried me, as I don't feel comfortable not being in full control.

Despite detailed explanation of what to expect in a hypnotic induction, that is learning how to achieve deep relaxation and heighten control over affec-tive/behavioural status and gut motility, patients assumed they would 'go under' meaning lose consciousness, e.g.

> Although I found the tapes relaxing, I struggled with the hypnotherapy, as I wasn't sure whether what I experienced was the full thing or not.

Although patients were apprehensive, their main reasons for participating included a desire for symptom improvement and/or a better understanding of IBS, e.g.

> I knew I wouldn't be cured but I felt I would learn more about IBS and bring my symptoms under control and perhaps not worry about them, which causes them to erupt.

With the exception of three participants, all patients reported that their hopes had been realized and their concerns adequately discussed within the groups.

COPING SKILLS, SYMPTOM CONTROL AND PATIENT SATISFACTION

The majority of respondents (72%) reported that the most helpful aspects of the programme were in meeting other IBS sufferers and sharing experiences, together with the insights gained from the therapeutic process. Typical vignettes illustrate:

> I thoroughly enjoyed it.... we were all connected in some way that helped us to share thoughts and emotions and help each other develop as 'normal' individuals in a society so ignorant of IBS.

> The self-awareness which developed, gave me a gradually growing understanding of how my thoughts and feelings were affecting my gut (something I had not previously acknowledged).

Almost all patients (98%) valued the therapists, e.g.

> I thought our therapist was excellent at managing the group dynamics and accurately pinpointing issues, which affected the different members. She presented the material clearly and effectively. I felt she understood what people were saying and where they were coming from.

Despite initial misconceptions about hypnotherapy, the majority (60%) favoured this approach, exemplified by a typical quotation:

> The most helpful aspects were the techniques such as self-hypnosis and visualization, which have encouraged me to seek a more 'active' role in controlling my gut habits.

A total of 40% preferred CBT. Patients demonstrated considerable comprehension of the cognitive model and how cognitive restructuring could help them cope with their various situations, e.g.

> The cognitive-behavioural therapy was the best part for me because it gave me valuable insights into the thought patterns, which fed my IBS and anxiety, plus some mental tools for changing my negative thoughts.

Behavioural assignment and stress management techniques were also appreciated. A typical vignette was:

> They helped me take control of my phobia, take more action to be more assertive with different aspects of my life.

Almost all (94%) found the supportive literature useful, e.g.

> I thought the literature was very useful in providing back up to what we had learned in the sessions.

The information regarding the effects of foods on the hypersensitive gut, coupled with the gradual introduction of more varied nutrition, liberated some patients (20%) from self-imposed restricted diets, e.g.

> I am now convinced that IBS is a mental/emotional problem not diet.

A small minority however (2%) found this advice unacceptable, e.g.

> It would be nice to have a dietician on hand.

A total of 64% of the sample enjoyed a walk provided by their group leader. The planned toilet stops and lunch break did much to increase confidence, illustrated by the following:

> *The company was lovely; I forgot all about my IBS, the day was relaxed and fun! fun! fun!*

> *I would have dreaded the thought of lunch in public a few months ago.... I haven't been on such a lovely walk since I was a child.*

Approximately 50% of the sample found the self-assessment (action plan) useful to clarify achievements, identify/solve problems, prioritize and set goals, e.g.

> *Writing things down helped me see clearly all the things I need to do to get the best out of what we have been learning and how to go about it.*

A total of 25% did not find the plan useful, e.g.

> *I didn't feel it was particularly helpful as my goals were constantly changing. My progress wasn't easy to record as the benefits were mainly emotional. I didn't have clear goals, more a general improvement in thought, mind and body.*

A total of 25% declined to comment. An example from those that did:

> *I often thought, what's the point of this exercise, but as the sessions progressed, the importance of the discussion became obvious. I now feel as though the whole process was necessary to get to this stage where I feel that I have control over my symptoms.*

Although some participants preferred certain aspects, many valued the programme as a whole.

Service improvement

Patients' perceptions of the least beneficial aspects of the programme and suggestions for improvement were as follows:

- Most concerns focussed on premises, which for 6% were too small, cold, noisy or uncomfortable
- Seven patients would have preferred more information on food intolerance and the medical aspects of IBS
- Three of the latter were unable to accept that psychological factors could influence their condition
- Ten found diary keeping and/or action plans difficult to complete
- Eight were uncomfortable with listening to the problems of others
- Four would have liked greater homogeneity in terms of condition, personal background and gender
- Three would have preferred individual therapy
- One patient did not like the therapist
- One patient found CBT counterproductive:

> *Why is it necessary to spend one third of the programme in discussion and dwelling on such abject negativity. After this I always felt most uncomfortable ... and consider the cognitive therapy to be counterproductive.*

Patients felt inhibited by the group member-led sessions, which were poorly attended. Participants were less likely to disclose in the absence of the therapist and thought these sessions lacked discipline. A typical quotation illustrates:

> *Nothing got done, we just talked. I didn't think that the group member-led sessions were necessary and it would have been far better to have a therapist-led group.*

The vast majority of respondents, however, reported that the programme could not be improved, expressed gratitude and the hoped that more patients could participate.

> *The programme was excellent. I can't imagine it being any better.*

> *I am grateful that I had the opportunity to join this self-help group. I know I will go from strength to strength in the future.*

> *The group approach is ... the answer to solving IBS for all sufferers, no matter how varied and different their symptoms may be. It should be extended to all counties.*

Therapists' views

The aim of therapists' feedback was to assess the efficacy of the manual and intervention from the practitioner's perspective. A thematic evaluation indicated that the therapists' views were consistent with those of the patients. The main themes identified were:

- Past/present trauma
- Reappraisal of thoughts and behaviours led to improvement in psychological and physical symptoms
- Therapist satisfaction and service improvements.

Past/present trauma

A great many psychological difficulties were elicited including physical/sexual abuse and other childhood/prior traumas. These issues were frequently associated with current or recent social stresses. Providing a safe environment for emotional expression led to subsequent insights into feelings and behaviours, e.g.

> *The session began with Audrey who had been rejected by her boyfriend. Audrey is unable to trust because of physical violence during her previous marriage. She was able to cry for the first time in 3 years.*

> *Geraldine said that stress and relationship problems triggered her IBS symptoms. Exploration of this statement revealed present difficulties with her adolescent son and a former troublesome relationship with her mother, both causing crippling guilt and subsequent approval-seeking behaviour.*

Patients felt misunderstood by the medical profession, e.g.

> *Many members felt they had no support from their doctors.*

Reappraisal of thoughts and behaviours

Reappraisal of thoughts and behaviours improved both psychological and physical health. There was much evidence of maladaptive coping, catastrophizing thinking and high social compliance, e.g.

Rob is so concerned with perfectionism he is afraid to paint his window frames in case the neighbours think it is not perfect.

Gill blames herself for losing a twin daughter at birth and the surviving twin being born handicapped. After a lengthy labour, the midwife told her 'she must hang on to her babies'. Cognitive exploration revealed a history of hypercritical parents. Consequently, Gill felt unable to go out without the child (now adult). Severe IBS and migraine gave her a reason to stay at home and care for her daughter.

The most important step forward ... was in their seeing clearly how psychological factors played such a crucial role in their IBS.

Breaking the cycle of negative automatic thoughts and maladaptive behaviour did much to reduce both anxiety and IBS symptoms. A typical report stated that:

Elizabeth reported an experience of being stuck in a commuter train for 45 min. In the recent past she would have suffered panic and diarrhoea but had been able to remain unconcerned which she said was 'fantastic'.

Simon had constant racing thoughts, a whole list of things he HAD to do. Isolating and challenging these thoughts made him realize that he doesn't have to do these things. In fact most of them were not important. Simon became more relaxed and his IBS symptoms greatly improved.

Members commented on how helpful they found the tapes and were making significant improvements through using them on a daily basis.

The hypnotherapy tapes were favourably commented on by 95% of therapists.

Therapist satisfaction

All therapists valued the manual and considered the programme effective.

All went according to plan from the word go. The group gelled quickly and the sessions fit appropriately into the 3 h.

I do have a sense of real satisfaction as I look back and a feeling of having been engaged in something that has been really worthwhile and therapeutically enhancing for all group members.

The only consistent problem associated with the manual was the group member-led sessions, e.g.

This session is marked as 'group member-led' but none of the group was inclined to come forward as a 'leader'. The feeling of this group, and a similar statement was expressed in my last group, that it is inappropriate/unnecessary to have group member-led sessions in the programme.

For five groups, therapists ran these sessions themselves or invited a colleague to facilitate them.

Hypno-psychotherapy for functional gastrointestinal disorders

Therapists found the action plan useful for less motivated patients, as it confronted them with their evasive behaviour, e.g.

'There was some laughter as I reminded them that if they had a fantasy of just coming along and being handed the Holy Grail, or given a magic wand to end all their problems, then it just wasn't like that. If they were not prepared to take risks and try something different, things would stay the same. I think they are getting the message.

Service improvement/patient dissatisfaction

A rash of drop-outs occurred in one group with new members recruited part way through the programme. None of the latter completed treatment causing concern to the therapist:

My concern over our low numbers put the group at risk. The 'new' members did not stay the course. Their late introduction threatened the safety of the group.

Some therapists reported that patients in receipt of incapacity benefit did not find the programme helpful. Therapists' commentary about financial benefits encompassed eight groups, e.g.

It struck me that, out of the four groups I ran, those patients on incapacity benefit failed to improve.

I have noticed that the group members who are on incapacity benefit, or who are not able to work because of their IBS, have not improved as much as the others. It's almost as though their 'illness' has become their identity.

Therapists felt that the most important consideration in this type of intervention was the patients' view of the cause of symptoms. Those unable to attribute their symptoms, at least in part to stress, did not profit from the intervention which supported former findings. Comparison studies have shown that patients who attribute their symptoms solely to physical disorder have a poorer medical treatment outcome than those willing to accept psychological influences (Bleijenberg & Fenin 1989, van Der Horst et al 1997). This was particularly true of food phobia. Most patients concerned with the influence of certain foods on their symptoms were greatly relieved by the explanation that it was the hypersensitivity of the gut that caused problems with food, and as the former became less sensitive with the therapeutic process, they were able to eat normally. For example:

Michael reported having had allergy tests done by several different 'experts' and all had provided different results. Most of his food intolerance disappeared following reduction of his symptoms.

Only a tiny minority (2%) retained their original belief in food intolerance and severely limited their diet. This was of grave concern to therapists, as patients were at risk from malnutrition with its attendant physical and psychological deterioration. A typical report states:

Julie has extreme food phobia, at one time eating only crackers, nothing else! She remains very defensive of her actions.

Three patients suffered an initial adverse reaction to hypnotherapy (unexpected cathartic release). These issues were explored and overcome in the therapeutic environment and, as such, were considered to be beneficial. The figures for abreaction are consistent with former findings (Finlay & Jones 1996).

On completion of the intervention, patients were encouraged to cascade their learned skills by attracting new members to their continuation support groups. This was ineffective and possibly even harmful. Out of the 158 patients who completed the programme, 100 opted to continue meeting as support groups or join existing support groups (63%). Collectively, these groups recruited 20 additional members without experience of the programme. Most support groups meet monthly and engage in a variety of activities such as discussion of IBS symptoms, personal problems, self-help strategies, guest speakers and social outings. A total of 64% however, withdrew after an average of two sessions, the one exception being an amalgamated group conducted by their former therapist and a gastrointestinal specialist nurse. The reason for this high attrition rate is generally unknown. However, one patient voiced the concerns of others who felt 'pressured' to attend an 'unnecessary' follow-up group:

It keeps you in IBS. I'm OK now, it's time to leave it behind.

The findings suggest that the combination of therapies provide advanced skills in coping with IBS and the low attrition rate (16%) implies that the programme was acceptable to most participants. Support from fellow patients was seen as an important factor and patients were able to describe how having the opportunity to talk about their feelings helped them. Fear of hypnotherapy and initial defensiveness associated with having a chronic debilitating condition in a society which trivializes functional somatic disorders, was quickly broken down by the therapeutic alliance. Taking the patients' very real symptoms seriously and providing a safe environment for emotional expression allowed subsequent insight into feelings and behaviour. This, together with the use of cognitive coping and restructuring strategies provided an alternative perspective to the patients' view of their personal situations, thus reducing the need for somatic expression. In line with former evidence that IBS patients tend to deny or minimize the effects of adverse life events (Toner et al 1990), many participants had formerly viewed their condition purely in physical terms and when under stress, tended to report somatic complaints and express concerns about their physical health. These findings support the large body of evidence suggesting that psychosocial factors mediate the intensity of IBS symptoms and illness behaviour and distinguish between treatment-seeking and non-treatment-seeking patients (Creed 1999, Douglas & Drossman 1999). Hypnotherapy was highly valued, particularly in relation to relaxation and exerting control over gut function. However, despite detailed assessment, an adverse reaction did occur in three patients, highlighting the necessity for hypnotherapy to be provided by appropriately trained practitioners in a contained environment. As the programme was originally designed for patient–graduate facilitation using autohypnosis tapes, this was a cause for re-evaluation.

Behavioural assignments such as activity scheduling and stress management were seen as useful tools in personal empowerment. Not only was the intervention appreciated but also patients valued the therapists

Hypno-psychotherapy for functional gastrointestinal disorders

themselves, supporting the widely held view that the therapeutic relationship is central to treatment outcome. The educational aspects of the programme and supporting literature were appreciated by almost all, as were the walks for those who participated (64%). Less popular elements included group member-led sessions and self-assessment procedures, with only 50% of the sample finding these aspects useful. Many patients failed to attend when the therapist was not present while others felt these sessions were unprofessional and inhibiting. Indeed, not all therapists complied with the manual in relation to lay leadership and facilitated these sessions themselves. Conversely, therapists felt that personal action planning motivated reluctant participants, and should be retained in a more user-friendly format supporting previous findings (Toner et al 1998). Similarly, some patients had initial difficulties with diary keeping, which is not uncommon in CBT.

Without exception, therapists found the intervention rewarding and valued the manual. The difficulties observed with participant-led groups raise questions about the significance of patient-led support groups. It may be that such groups offer respite from compromised doctor–patient relationships. The reluctance of patients to facilitate these sessions and their disinclination to join/remain in future lay-led support groups, cautiously suggests that engaging in such activities conflicts with their changing/positive perceptions acquired through the therapeutic process. These findings suggest that the intervention should be entirely therapist-led and formally ended after the final session.

The therapists' observations regarding the small minority who were unable to profit from the intervention have implications for assessment. Patients incapable of psychological insight tend to experience emotional distress almost exclusively in physical symptoms and are particularly hypervigilant to the stigma associated with psychological explanations (Toner et al 1998). In the present study, this was particularly pertinent to those unable to relinquish food phobia. In contrast to an earlier study (Houghton et al 1996), some therapists reported that patients, in receipt of state incapacity benefits, failed to improve. This may reflect financial concerns, preventing patients from responding to the programme. More recent work (Taylor et al 2005, Taylor 2007) has found that if employment-related anxiety is explored and resolved, it can lead to a healthy return to work. For the vast majority, however, the programme represented a successful treatment package, strengthening existing evidence for the provision of psychological interventions in IBS. To reduce costs, the intervention has since been reduced to an eight-session professionally led programme.

SUMMARY

This chapter has discussed IBS and functional dyspepsia, which make up the largest group of FGID. A vicious circle of misunderstanding has resulted from the traditional diagnosis of exclusion. The last three decades have witnessed research leading to the growing awareness that such conditions result from biological, psychosocial and environmental factors. As such treatment should encompass the whole patient rather than just the physical aspects. Published work demonstrating the clinical efficacy of dynamic psychotherapy, CBT and hypnotherapy has been outlined. Differing opinions as to how GDHT exerts its benefits have been presented but overall this body of literature suggests that psychosocial interventions should be routinely available for IBS. This raises the question of appropriate training for medical personnel. Time constraints and disinclination to address the psychosocial factors associated with FGID can compromise doctor–patient relationships. A national study has assessed the feasibility of the provision of professionally and lay-led combined group CBT and hypnotherapy in IBS, and a qualitative investigation has added further insight into participants' and therapists' experiences of the treatment process. While lay-led support groups failed to maintain recruitment, the therapist-led groups demonstrated significant improvements in both GI and psychosocial symptoms and the scheme was highly valued by participants.

RECOMMENDATIONS FOR EDUCATION, TRAINING AND DEVELOPMENT

Medical and other personnel involved in caring for patients with FGID need to have the ability to elicit patients' key concerns within a time-limited consultation. This is currently included in the curriculum for training medical students but there is no requirement for existing doctors (other than those caring for cancer patients) to undergo this training. An evidence-based 3-day training course in Advanced Communication Skills for senior health professionals could easily be adapted for general use (National Cancer Action Team 2008).

A further recommendation would be the availability of centres providing specialist psychological therapies for this patient population. At the time of writing, only three such centres exist in England (London, South Manchester and East Lancashire). The latter receives Primary Care Trust (PCT) funding but patients can only be referred from consultants, which is a bone of contention for GPs. Although hypnotherapy is now recommended by NICE, all referrals must be individually approved by the appropriate PCT. These referral methods perpetuate the diagnosis of exclusion, excessive treatment-seeking behaviour and increased healthcare costs. It is therefore suggested that the Rome criteria should be included in the training of all personnel who care for patients with FGID and for those responsible for healthcare budgets.

Subject to funding, an eight-session combined group CBT, hypnotherapy and education programme is available for national dissemination. Training in psychological approaches in the management of IBS is also available for appropriately qualified personnel. (Training and provision costs are available on request for REAL Wellbeing at: www.realtd.co.uk.)

ACKNOWLEDGEMENTS

The author is grateful to the National Lottery for supporting the feasibility study and to the research participants.

Barabasz, A., Barabasz, M., 2006. Effects of tailored and manualized hypnotic inductions for complicated irritable bowel syndrome patients. Int. J. Clin. Exp. Hypn. 54 (1), 100–112.

Beck, A.T., 1993. Cognitive therapy: nature and relation to behaviour therapy. J. Psychother. Pract. Res. 2 (4), 342–356.

Bleijenberg, G., Fenin, J.F.M., 1989. Anamnestic and psychologic features in diagnosis and prognosis of functional abdominal complaints: a prospective study. Gut 30, 1076–1081.

Clark, C., DeLegge, M., 2008. Irritable bowel syndrome: a practical approach. Nutr. Clin. Pract. 33 (3), 263–267.

Creed, F., 1999. The relationship between psychosocial parameters and outcome in irritable bowel syndrome. Am. J. Med. 107 (5A), 74s–80s.

Creed, F., Fernandes, I., Guthrie, E., et al., 2003. The cost-effectiveness of psychotherapy and paroxetine for severe irritable bowel syndrome. Gastroenterology 124, 303–317.

Douglas, A., Drossman, M.D., 1999. Do psychosocial factors define symptom severity and patient status in irritable bowel syndrome? Am. J. Med. 107 (5A), 41s–50s.

Drossman, D.A., Li, Z., Andruzzi, E., et al., 1993. US Householder survey of functional gastrointestinal disorders. Prevalence, sociodemography and health impact. Dig. Dis. Sci. 38, 1569–1580.

Drossman, D.A., Toner, B.B., Whitehead, W.E., et al., 2003. Cognitive-behavioral therapy versus education and desipramine versus placebo for moderate to severe functional bowel disorders. Gastroenterology 125 (1), 19–31.

Finlay, I.G., Jones, O.L., 1996. Hypnotherapy in palliative care. J. R. Soc. Med. 89, 493–496.

Greene, B., Blanchard, E.B., 1994. Cognitive therapy for irritable bowel syndrome. J. Consult. Clin. Psychol. 62 (3), 576–582.

Gonsalkorale, W.M., Houghton, L.A., Whorwell, P.J., 2002. Hypnotherapy in irritable bowel syndrome: a large-scale audit of a clinical service examination of factors influencing responsiveness. Am. J. Gastroenterol. 97 (4), 954–961.

Gonsalkorale, W.M., Miller, V., Afzal, A., et al., 2003. Long-term benefits of hypnotherapy for irritable bowel syndrome. Gut 52 (11), 1623–1629.

Gonsalkorale, W.M., Toner, B.B., Whowell, P.J., 2004. Cognitive change in patients undergoing hypnotherapy for irritable bowel syndrome. Psychosom. Res. 56 (3), 271–278.

Guthrie, E., Creed, F., Dawson, D., et al., 1991. A controlled trial of psychological treatment for the irritable bowel syndrome. Gastroenterology 100, 450–457.

Haines, A., Jones, R., 1994. Implementing findings of research. Br. J. Med. 308, 1488–1492.

Harvey, R.F., Hinton, R.A., Gunary, R.M., et al., 1989. Individual and group hypnotherapy in the treatment of refractory irritable bowel syndrome. Lancet 1, 424–425.

Heaton, K., Thompson, W.G., 1999. The irritable bowel syndrome: a critique. Gastroenterology 95, 232–241.

Hendler, C.S., Redd, W.H., 1986. Fear of hypnosis: the role of labelling in patients' acceptance of behavioural interventions. Behav. Ther. 17, 2–13.

Houghton, L.A., Heyman, D.J., Whorwell, P.J., 1996. Symptomatology, quality of life and economic features of irritable bowel syndrome: the effect of hypnotherapy. Aliment. Pharmacol. Ther. 10, 91–95.

Jones, P., Crowel, M., Olden, K.W., et al., 2007. Functional gastrointestinal disorders: an update for the psychiatrist. Psychosomatics 48, 93–102.

Kirsch, I., Montgomery, G., Sapirstein, G., 1995. Hypnosis as an adjunct to cognitive-behavioural psychotherapy, a meta-analysis. J. Consult. Clin. Psychol. 63, 214–220.

Koutsomanis, D., 1997. Hypoanalgesia in the irritable bowel syndrome. Gastroenterology 112, A764.

Lackner, J.M., Mesmer, C., Morley, S., et al., 2004. Psychological treatments for irritable bowel syndrome: a systematic review and meta-analysis. J. Consult. Clin. Psychol. 72 (6), 1100–1113.

Lackner, J.M., Jaccard, J., Krasner, S.S., et al., 2007. How does cognitive behaviour therapy for irritable bowel syndrome work? A mediational analysis of a randomized clinical trial. Gastroenterology 133 (2), 702–705.

Lea, R., Houghton, L.A., Calver, E.L., et al., 2003. Gut focussed hypnotherapy normalizes disordered rectal sensitivity inpatients with irritable bowel syndrome. Aliment. Pharmacol. Ther. 17 (5), 635–642.

Levy, R.L., Olden, K.W., Nalliboff, B.D., et al., 2006. Psychosocial aspects of the functional gastrointestinal disorders. Gastroenterology 130 (5), 1447–1458.

National Cancer Action Team, 2008. National Advanced Communication Skills Training Programme for senior health professionals in cancer care. London Strategic Health Authority, London.

Neff, D.F., Blanchard, E.B., 1987. A multicomponent treatment for irritable bowel syndrome. Behav. Ther. 18, 70–83.

NICE (National Institute for Health and Clinical Excellence), 2008. Irritable bowel syndrome in adults: diagnosis and management of the irritable bowel syndrome in primary care. Department of Health, London.

Palsson, O.S., Turner, M.J., Johnson, D.A., et al., 2002. Hypnosis treatment for severe irritable bowel syndrome: investigation of mechanism and effects on symptoms. Dig. Dis. Sci. 47 (11), 2605–2614.

Payne, A., Blanchard, E.B., 1995. A controlled comparison of cognitive therapy and self-help support groups in the treatment of irritable bowel syndrome. J. Consult. Clin. Psychol. 63 (5), 779–786.

Sandler, R.S., 1990. Epidemiology of irritable bowel syndrome in the United States. Gastroenterology 99, 409–414.

Schoenberger, N.E., 2000. Research on hypnosis as an adjunct to cognitive-behavioural psychotherapy. Int. J. Clin. Exp. Hypn. 48, 154–169.

SF-36, 2001. Physical and mental health summary scales: a manual for users. Online. Available:www.qualitymetric.com.

Simren, M., Ringstrom, G., Bjornsson, E.S., et al., 2004. Treatment with hypnotherapy reduces the sensory and motor component of the gastrocolonic response in irritable bowel syndrome. Psychosom. Med. 66, 233–238.

Spiller, R.C., 2005. Irritable bowel syndrome. Br. Med. Bull. 72, 15–29.

Talley, N.J., Gabriel, S.E., Harmesen, W.S., et al., 1995. Medical costs in community subjects with irritable bowel syndrome. Gastroenterology 109, 1736–1741.

Taylor, E.E., 2007. Group cognitive-behaviour therapy in the management of chronic incapacity: participants' views. Unpublished evaluation, available from liz.taylor@realtd.co.uk.

Taylor, E.E., Read, N.W., Hills, H.M., 2004a. Combined group cognitive-behaviour therapy and hypnotherapy in the management of the irritable bowel syndrome: the feasibility of clinical provision. Behavioural and Cognitive Psychotherapy 32, 99–106.

Taylor, E.E., Read, N.W., Hills, H.M., 2004b. Combined group cognitive-behaviour therapy and hypnotherapy in the management of the irritable bowel syndrome: A qualitative evaluation of patients' and therapists' views. Unpublished evaluation, available fromliz.taylor@realtd.co.uk.

Taylor, E.E., Hewitt, M.P., Platt, C.J., et al., 2005. Group cognitive-behaviour therapy in the management of chronic incapacity. Presented at the North West Public Health Conference: 'Public health delivery moving it forward', Southport, Merseyside 19/20th April.

Thompson, G., 2006. The road to Rome. Gastroenterology 130, 1552–1556.

Toner, B.B., 2005. Cognitive-behavioural therapy treatment of irritable bowel syndrome. CNS Spectr. 10 (11), 883–890.

Toner, B.B., Garfinkle, P.E., Jeejeebhoy, K.N., et al., 1990. Self-schema in irritable bowel syndrome and depression. Psychosom. Med. 52, 149–155.

Toner, B.B., Segal, Z.V., Emmot, S., et al., 1998. Cognitive-behavioural group therapy for patients with irritable bowel syndrome. Int. J. Group Psychother. 48 (2), 215–243.

van Der Horst, H.E., Van Dulmen, A.M., Schellevis, F.G., et al., 1997. Do patients with irritable bowel syndrome in primary care really differ from outpatients with irritable bowel syndrome? Gut 41, 669–674.

Van Dulmen, A.M., Fennis, J., Bleijenberg, G., 1996. Cognitive-behavioural group therapy for irritable bowel syndrome: effects and long-term follow up. Psychosom. Med. 58, 508–514.

Vlieger, A.M., Menko-Frankenhuis, C., Wolfkamp, S.C., et al., 2007. Hypnotherapy for children with functional abdominal pain or irritable bowel syndrome: a randomized controlled trial. Gastroenterology 133 (5), 1430–1436.

Whitehead, E.W., 2006. Hypnosis for irritable bowel syndrome: the empirical evidence of therapeutic effects. Int. J. Clin. Exp. Hypn. 54 (1), 7–20.

Hypno-psychotherapy for functional gastrointestinal disorders

Whorwell, P.J., Prior, A., Faragher, E.B., 1984. Controlled trial of hypnotherapy in the treatment of severe refractory irritable bowel syndrome. Lancet 1232–1233.

Whorwell, P.J., Prior, A., Colgan, S.M., 1987. Hypnotherapy in severe irritable bowel syndrome: further experience. Gut 28, 423–425.

Whorwell, P.J., Houghton, L.A., Taylor, E.E., et al., 1992. Physiological effects of emotion: Assessment via hypnosis. Lancet 340, 69–72.

Whorwell, P.J., 2009. Hypnotherapy for irritable bowel syndrome: the response of colonic and non-colonic symptoms. J. Psychosom. Res. 64 (6), 621–623.

Wilson, S., Maddison, T., Roberts, L., et al., 2006. Systematic review: the effectiveness of hypnotherapy in the management of irritable bowel syndrome. Aliment. Pharmacol. Ther. 24 (5), 769.

USEFUL RESOURCES

REAL Wellbeing, St James Centre, 8 St James Square, Bacup, Lancashire OL13 9AA. Tel: 01706 871730; e-mail: info@realtd.co.uk; website: www.realtd.co.uk.

The Register of Approved Gastrointestinal Psychotherapists and Hypnotherapists. First Floor, 18 Carr Road, Nelson, Lancashire BB9 7JS. Tel: 0800 161 3823/ 01282 716839; e-mail: admin@nrhp.co.uk; website: www.nrhp.co.uk.

Existential hypnotherapy in life-threatening illness

Anne Cawthorn • Bernadette Shepherd • Kevin Dunn • Peter A. Mackereth

CHAPTER CONTENTS

CHAPTER OUTLINE

One of the most rewarding, yet challenging areas, for a therapist, is working with patients who are coming to terms with their own mortality. This chapter explores key therapeutic issues for therapists working with existential anxiety. Being with a person who is facing a life-threatening illness reminds us all of our own mortality and provides opportunities to give the best of ourselves in our work. In the spirit of recognizing that we are merely companions at this time, honoured by the invitation from patients and their carers to provide care and support, we introduce the **SERVICE** model.

© 2010 Elsevier Ltd.
DOI: 10.1016/B978-0-7020-3082-6.00016-2

KEY WORDS

Existential
Anxiety
SERVICE Model
Spirituality
Companion

INTRODUCTION

Supporting someone who is experiencing an existential crisis requires high levels of personal and professional development. This work is never easy, as it requires us to look at our own personal vulnerability, reminding us that we too are mortal. Kearney (2000) says that to fear death is neither a sign of weakness nor a reason for shame; it is part of what makes us alive and human. Dame Cicely Saunders (1995) founder of the hospice movement, further suggests that what we learn from the challenge of working with the dying, helps us on both a personal and professional level; because it teaches us to avoid our professional mask, and learn the skill of just being 'person to person' in the depths of their pain.

The rewards associated with this area of work come when we are invited by the patient to be a companion on their special journey. Just as birthing is greatly assisted by a competent midwife, likewise, facing one's own mortality and/or impending death, can be facilitated by a competent therapist or healthcare professional (HCP) who is willing to walk alongside someone. Many feel unprepared to do this. However, experienced palliative care professionals all suggest that we should let the patient be our teachers when we journey with them, as this will teach us as much about living as about dying (Kearney 2000, Kubler-Ross 1997, Saunders 1995). The notion of the companion will be explored throughout this chapter using existential literature, along with the experiences of the authors, who have been privileged to walk alongside patients, as companions on their existential journey. When reflecting on these experiences, by working in this way, death has become less of a stranger to us, and more of a familiar acquaintance.

EXISTENTIAL THEORY

Existentialism (from the Danish and German term *Existenz*) is the philosophy concerned with the subjective, personal dimension of human existence in terms of the existing individual (Honderich 1995). It describes the distinctively human mode of being, the ontological 'givens' of existence and the clarification of what it means to be alive (Deurzen-Smith 1995). The Danish writer and social critic Soren Kierkegaard (1813–1855) discussed how human existence is essentially one of anxiety, set with tension between the finite and infinite. Thus, the challenge of living is to find a balance between possibility and necessity and in the process, become 'true' to oneself, i.e. through being self determining (Kierkegaard 1844).

The German philosopher, Heidegger (1927), is most often regarded as the founder of Existentialism. He used the word *Dasein* to denote as 'human being' the kind of being for whom 'being' or existence raises all sorts of questions and issues (Inwood 1997). This 'human being' 'Dasein', also entails a number of other concepts such as being-in-the-world and being-towards-death. In other words, being human always involves living within a particular set of circumstances, having a particular past and looking towards a particular future. Resolutely to face these facts and to live with them is to live authentically (Inwood 1997). By contrast 'inauthenticity' is seen as a defence against the anxiety of this realization and is marked by a resignation to convention, conformity and duty, i.e. by doing what people imagine is expected of them (Deurzen-Smith 1988).

According to Heidegger (1927), the most fundamental philosophical questions are: 'why is there something rather than nothing?' and 'what is the meaning of being?' We do not actually know the answer to these questions, but most people sooner or later ask them; especially when diagnosed with a life-threatening illness. Drawing upon an existential hypnotherapy approach to our work, allows for the patient to confront and clarify the meaning of their diagnosis and the underlying related anxiety, rather than just attempt to reduce or eliminate it. As an attempt to undertake a complete overview of existential theory is beyond the scope of this text, the authors intend to describe some of the major existential principles, which theoretically and philosophically underpin the psycho-hypnotherapy clinical work discussed in this chapter.

THE MEANING OF EXISTENTIAL ANXIETY

The experience of meaninglessness and the creation of meaning are closely related to the experience of angst or existential anxiety. King and Citrenbaum (1993: 16) argue that this existential anxiety occurs against the backdrop of the personal realization that 'I am alone in the world and I have to contend with my mortality, and other limitations, by taking responsibility for myself in the face of endless challenges and confusions'. When therapists work existentially, they concern themselves with the 'givens' of human existence which are: death, anxiety, meaningless, isolation, choice, freedom and responsibility and how these are negotiated (or not). This is undertaken through the interpretations and meanings given to the experience of self, others, and the world, and how in turn, this shapes our sense of reality (Deurzen-Smith 1988). As such, it regards that all people's forms of human dilemma, tragedy and suffering are fundamentally problems about 'being in the world'. Spinelli (1989) argues that as a result, all patients difficulties are seen to reflect their attempts to avoid, resist or deny the angst and uncertainty that authentic living demands.

Existentialists see anxiety as a 'calling card to the future' (King & Citrenbaum 1993: 16). They report that people are addicted to emotional safety in today's uncertain world; and go on to argue that to be attached to emotional safety is to be attached to the illusion of psychological safety. A diagnosis of a life-threatening illness challenges the average person to move away from the sameness of everyday life, and the accompanying anxiety becomes the cue for that person to want to flee back to sameness and when this is not possible, anxiety increases.

The therapeutic encounter can be regarded as an invitation for the patient to explore the meaning of their anxiety, which often arises as a result of their diagnosis. Patients need to be encouraged to move forward in the face of anxiety and therefore need to be supported and congratulated for every small step they take. Working existentially involves teaching patients to manage their reactions to anxiety.

The key to effective existential hypnosis is the therapist–patient dialogue; in particular what is communicated about hypnosis and what is communicated during hypnosis. Hypnotherapy techniques can teach patients to reduce their anxiety to a manageable level (see below). King and Citrenbaum (1993: 17) argue that the aim of therapy is to never totally eliminate the feeling of anxiety, because that would doom the therapy to failure: as death is the only total anxiety reducer life has to offer. They go on to suggest that learning to be anxious in the right way, not too much or too little, is the key to living a reflective, meaningful human life and adjusting to a life-threatening illness. Kierkegaard (1844: 155) said that 'whoever has learnt to be anxious in the right way has learnt the ultimate'.

WORKING WITH EXISTENTIAL ISSUES

Working with an existential crisis, the therapist needs to give the patient permission to share and work with their existential concerns and gain the patient's permission to use hypnotherapy techniques.

This requires the following three factors:

1. The therapist needs to be comfortable and personally prepared to work in this way
2. Be able to develop and use the therapeutic relationship
3. Elicit the source of their existential concerns/anxiety and utilize a range of hypnotherapeutic approaches.

PERSONAL PREPARATION OF THE THERAPIST

For the therapist to be a potent practitioner, it is essential that they have undergone personal preparation enabling them to be comfortable listening to, and discussing issues relating to death and dying. Patients soon pick up on whether therapists are 'big enough' to cope with their unspoken fears. Fear of dying is very common and Rinpoche (1998: 187) suggests that the deepest reason that we are afraid of death is possibly because we do not know who we are. He goes on to remind us that being with someone who is dying 'makes us poignantly aware not only of their mortality, but of our own'. It is important therefore, that before working in this way, the therapist needs to have addressed issues relating to their own mortality and have worked through personal fears about dying. Personal growth for the therapist should come about through processing thoughts and feelings about their mortality, utilizing personal therapy, supervision and ongoing training.

Neimeyer (1994) studied the concept of death anxiety and found that it is generally present in the normal population, and not just when there is an immediate threat to one's life. Neimeyer identified that there are 25 individual fears relating to death; these ranged from fear about being alone, fears relating to suffering, being in pain, and death being the end of everything. With this in mind, the therapist needs to ascertain what the patient's individual fear(s) is/are and what impact this has on them. They also need to be aware of their own personal anxiety in relation to death and be aware of how this impacts on their work with patients.

A diagnosis of cancer, or any other life-threatening illness, can leave the patient feeling that their world has been torn apart, resulting in personal suffering as they perceive their impending destruction (Cassell 1991). As patients face their existential crisis, an amount of anxiety is to be expected (Barraclough 1999). Learning to work with anxiety is important, while also recognizing that it may be accompanied by fear. Kearney (1997) suggests that fear for patients facing their own mortality can occur for a number of reasons; it may be linked to anticipation of physical pain and distress, emotional pain relating to separation from those they love, and dependency and loss of control, which they imagine, lies ahead. When faced with this crisis, a patient's natural reaction is to try to find ways of gaining some control and search for understanding.

Existential crises can relate to spirituality. Walter (1997) linked spirituality with a personal search for purpose and meaning. A study by Narayanasamy (1996) identified that an intense spiritual awakening could potentially be identified when patients are diagnosed with a chronic and life-threatening illness, as it is a pivotal life event. This leads patients to begin asking questions such as, 'Why me?', 'Why now?' and many others. The important lesson for both the therapist and the patient is that generally there are no answers to these questions. However, having the opportunity to share these questions should never be underestimated, along with having another person empathize with their dilemma. By connecting to another and having their questions heard, validated and normalized can in itself be extremely powerful. Cunningham (2000) shares this view saying that 'connectedness' is the route to healing.

If the person has someone to share their concerns with, it prevents them from feeling isolated and alone. Kearney (2000) suggests that if patients split off from parts of themselves and from others, fear and meaninglessness will continue to dominate for these vulnerable individuals. This is why the person who is struggling and suffering with the burden of illness and the uncertainty of their mortal life will require attendance to their whole experience of living and dying. The temptation to split mind, body and spirit can cause problems in existential care and although the therapist may have a strong driver to 'fix things' for patients on a variety of levels; including emotionally, physically and even spiritually, it is best to resist our initial urge to rush in and rescue, because through working together and paying attention to the whole, the answers will emerge.

Being curious

One way of working with a seriously ill or dying patient who is asking questions related to the meaning of life and death involves simply being curious, i.e. being actively interested in that person's life, their views and their questions. However, when a patient begins to talk about matters of life and death, these are not actual questions to be answered; rather it is the opening gambit of a conversation in which the patient is wrestling to find his or her own meaning. The purpose of this kind of 'curiosity' is to support, not prejudge or to lead the patient's process of discovery or uncovering of meaning. The language patients use is often of the cultural, religious and spiritual and the therapist can be curious about an individual's examination of their existence. If this is an unfamiliar situation, then the therapist may initially question his/her abilities to be present and interactive with a patient, who is in a sense testing or signalling their own quest.

People experienced in the use of curiosity as a technique offer the following: Mindell (2003: 37) suggests that curiosity is about having the skill to 'notice what we are experiencing, which feelings are occurring in any given moment' and 'what is driving the quest to gain understanding of the person's journey.' Johns (2004) recommends that this state of open curiosity requires a level of mindfulness, coupled with the knowledge that support exists, to enable them to reflect and process the experience, without becoming overwhelmed. This is where the therapist provides skilled companionship to the patient. Box 14.1 gives a Model, which represents this way of working.

The journey

The notion of journeying with the person is becoming the model, which has the potential to facilitate healing with this client group. Cassidy (1988) proposes a model of care in which both therapist and client are stripped of their roles, skills, techniques and all the paraphernalia of care, and relate to each other in a radically simple human-to-human way. Campbell (1994) by contrast, suggests that the therapist journeys with the patient as a skilled companion. He further suggests that the relationship is committed, but has clear boundaries, which are for the protection of both the practitioner and patient. It requires respect and even reverence towards the beliefs of others, e.g. working with and accepting the patient's values and beliefs, even when they may be at odds with our own. Campbell emphasizes the relationship should be on mutuality rather than risk going down the route of imposing expertise.

It is akin to Bion's (1962) definition of containment, which involves 'being there' with another in their suffering. A way of describing the different ways the therapist works when they become a companion to the patient, while

---

BOX 14.1 Model of spiritual care that encompasses SERVICE

Serving mindfully
Empathy and being open to the other
Respect beliefs
Valuing the person's way of being
Investment in the relationship recognizing that it is a journey of brief companionship
Curiosity about the other's and our own spiritual journey
Engagement but not engaged to an outcome.

they are on their own arduous existential voyage, is in the poem *Footprints* by Margaret Fishback Powers (1993):

> *A true companion will be strong enough to accompany them, staying in step.*

However, at times the following may also apply:

> *During your trials and testings, when you saw one set of footprints it was then that I carried you.*

A competent therapist will be able to evaluate whether their role as companion requires two sets of footprints or whether, on occasions only one set will be present.

DEVELOPING AND USING THE THERAPEUTIC RELATIONSHIP

A good therapeutic relationship is an essential pre-requisite for all therapy. However, when utilizing hypnotherapy techniques in challenging situations such as these, it is even more important. Erskine et al (1999) remind us that when the relationship is nurtured and entered into fully, it has the potential to be a vehicle for growth and healing. A number of authors suggest that when working with existential and spiritual domains, therapists should adopt a special relationship, which matches and mirrors the needs of the patient. Clarkson (1992) calls this the transpersonal relationship, which relates to the psychology of the soul and is potentially present in all healing encounters. It involves supporting patients to come to terms with existential threats linked to their own mortality. Cawthorn (2006) refers to it as the soulful relationship (Box 14.2) and goes on to describe a further relationship, which she calls the uncovered relationship, which the therapist uses when working with the unconscious.

Soul pain

When patients are diagnosed with a life-threatening illness, it is often psychologically painful. Kearney (1997) refers to the suffering experienced by patients facing their own mortality as 'soul pain'. He uses 'soul' in the more classical sense, referring to the 'psyche' and suggests that what occurs at this

---

BOX 14.2 The emergent relationship model

- *The Now Relationship* – working as partners in an adult-to-adult relationship
- *The Wanting Relationship* – where the therapist is aware that the client is vulnerable or needy, i.e. the therapist may be aware that they are not working as adult to adult, but like a nurturing parent to child
- *The Evoked Relationship* – involves transference and counter transference and somatized feelings are utilized in the work
- *The Soulful Relationship* – often clients who are coming to terms with a life-threatening or life-limiting illness begin to consider their own mortality
- *The Uncovered Relationship* – the therapist is either presented with, or deliberately chooses to use information gained from the patient's subconscious.

(From Cawthorn 2006. Working with the denied body.)

time is that the soul becomes vulnerable and suffers. To reach the psyche the therapist needs to access the right hand side of the brain using intuition, symbol, imagery and myth (Kearney 2000). Working with the soul is through working at a deeper level; through creating an environment which best facilitates the process of inner healing. This aligns with the uncovered relationship (Box 14.2) where the therapist works with the patient's unconscious, using hypnotherapy techniques, dream work, art therapy, music therapy, bodywork and/or mindful meditation. Using these approaches assists patients who are facing a life-threatening illness, and for whom logic sometimes needs to be suspended.

Personality

Each person's experience of illness and suffering has a unique meaning, expressing something of the individuality of the person who is having the experience (Seigal 2001). Studies into patients' personal individual adjustment styles, has led many to question whether this information can be used, to assess how they might adapt to illness or times of existential crisis (Wells 2001). Barraclough (1999) asserts that adjustment requires more than one approach. It requires supporting the patient to work through the losses they are facing, as well as working to dissolve some of the defence mechanisms, which are proving to be unhealthy (Box 14.3).

ELICIT THE SOURCE OF EXISTENTIAL ANXIETY AND UTILIZE A RANGE OF HYPNOTHERAPEUTIC APPROACHES

Before utilizing any hypnotherapy techniques, it is important to elicit information relating to the cause of the patient's existential anxiety. However, for some patients this information is not available in their conscious mind and

---

BOX 14.3 Case study 1

Tracy, a 38-year-old woman presented for therapy. She was approaching the terminal stage of her metastatic breast cancer. She was frightened about how she might die; worried about dying in pain and feeling isolated from her caring family. When exploring her normal coping style, it became clear that she had difficulty asking for support and showing vulnerability. This was leading her to feel anxious and out of control. Therapy with Tracy was to help her to adjust to her mortality, as she discounted the significance of it both for herself and for her family, and to find ways of gaining control. Using hypnotherapy, the source of the isolation was elicited. While in trance, Tracey accessed a brick wall, which she had erected around herself, as a form of protection. Through dialoguing with it, she inquired what purpose it was serving her. She soon realized that it was not helpful and indeed was the cause of her isolation. Through negotiation, Tracy was able to feel comfortable to take it down brick by brick. Her control issues related to her fear about dying which was resolved through discussion with her palliative care consultant and Tracy agreed to end-of-life care within the hospice (if necessary), in order to achieve good pain and symptom control.

can potentially be accessed via the unconscious using imagery. For patients who are comfortable using images, this is a wonderful way of visualizing something in the unconscious, which is not readily accessible to the conscious brain. Imagery goes on at all times in all individuals, both at a conscious and unconscious and maybe even the cellular level (Davis Brigham 1996). An important starting point in assessing suitability would be to explore the imagery already in place in relation to disease, health, values, fears and what the person sees as occurring in the body. Any guided imagery must be syntonic with the individual's core beliefs and it needs to fit in with their deepest values and not be contradictory with their view of the world. Cunningham (2000) suggests using two modes of imagery: 'diagnostic' and 'therapeutic'.

Diagnostic imagery

Diagnostic imagery is used either just to elicit information, or to form the basis from which the therapist can work with patients, using hypnotherapy techniques. The diagnostic use of mental imagery has a long history and goes back to the use of healing dreams by the ancient Greeks and Egyptians. Cunningham (2000) asserts that the central concept of this is that people access, in their imagery, ideas not readily available to the rational mind. An example of using diagnostic imagery is where the therapist invites the patient, while in trance, to explore what they see inside (or outside) their body. To notice the colours, textures, what they feel like and notice whether they would like to change anything. Many people are surprised by the information this gives them and are usually amenable to move on to the second mode of imagery.

Therapeutic imagery

Cunningham (2000) believes that the use of therapeutic imagery is an extension of the observation that images affect body function. The therapist through working in this way, encourages the patient to imagine beneficial changes in the images they have (see Box 14.4 and Ch. 6). Working in trance, the therapist needs to find out the patient's preferred way of working, whether it is an aggressive imagery such as 'zapping' their disease, or a more healing imagery, such as using a healing light, or 'magic' fluid.

BOX 14.4 Case study 2

An example of working in this way is with Jane who was a 44-year-old woman with extensive metastatic cancer in her lungs and liver from a primary bowel cancer. Using hypnotherapy we worked with the image she drew of her cancer. Figure 14.1 represented her image of her body and Figure 14.2 was the image of the cancer in her lung. I invited her, while in trance, to go inside and change anything she wanted to by drinking 'magic' healing fluid. This is a symbol drama technique, which is part of Leuner's (1969) GAI technique. This non-aggressive healing technique aligned with Jane's way of working and allowed her to clear away all the central brown and black images in Figure 14.1 and clear the black in Figure 14.2.

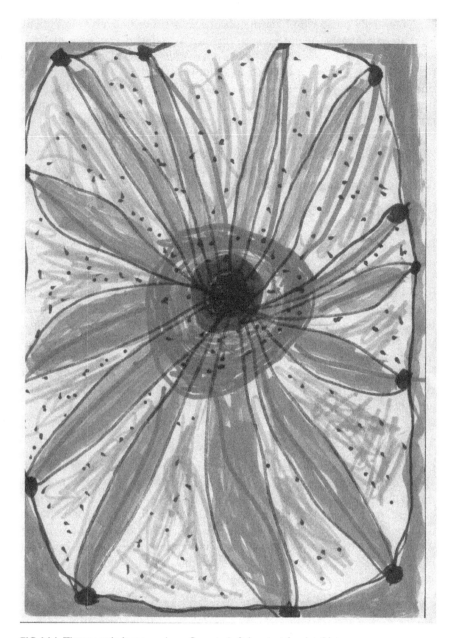

FIG 14.1 Therapeutic imagery. Jane, Case study 2 (see text for details).

DEPRESSION, ANXIETY AND ADJUSTMENT PROBLEMS

Before offering hypnotherapy techniques it is useful to screen the patient for symptoms of depression, anxiety or an adjustment disorder. These are common in this client group and respond well to hypnotherapy and cognitive-behavioural approaches. Depression is a much more common problem than most people appreciate. Yapko (2001) cites the 1999 WHO proclamation,

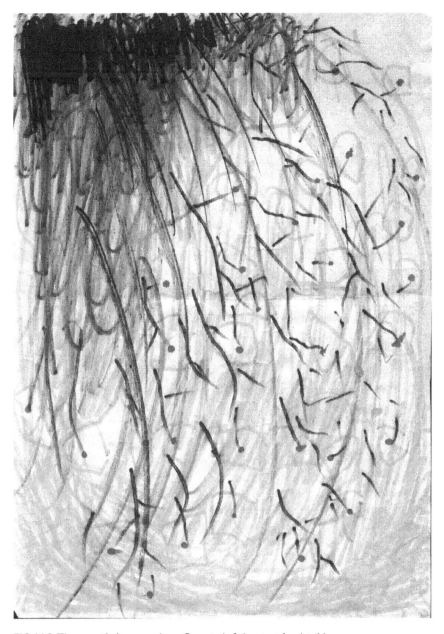

FIG 14.2 Therapeutic imagery. Jane, Case study 2 (see text for details).

which said that depression is the world's fourth most debilitating human condition, behind heart disease, cancer and traffic accidents. One in six of the general population suffer from depression in their lifetime, while in relation to people with a chronic illness, this figure rises significantly and is estimated to be anywhere between 25% with a cancer diagnosis rising to 50% when the person has a terminal diagnosis (NICE 2004).

If the mood is very low and the patient has suicidal thoughts or ideation, the therapist needs to refer back to the doctor for assessment, consideration of appropriate medication and/or support from the mental health team. Also assessing whether mood links with coping styles, such as helplessness, hopelessness, or avoidance, anxious preoccupation or loss of fighting spirit. In addition, the therapist must ascertain whether the patient has suppressed emotions, such as anger, guilt, despair, or fear, due to a perceived loss of control. Yapko (2001: 105–108), presents a framework in which he explores options within trance to help clients 'who are feeling "stuck"' to actively make both emotionally and intellectually intelligent decisions in relation to how that might work using hypnotherapy.

Anxiety is very common with this client group. This can be existential anxiety, acute distress and/or generalized anxiety, which may include phobia and panic. It is important therefore, to be able to assess the level of anxiety patients are experiencing and to work with them in ways which will either reduce it, or alternatively to be present with them, in feeling, and experiencing their anxiety. Hypnotherapy techniques, which help patients to reduce physical pain, such as use of a dial or anaesthetic glove technique can also help to reduce anxiety (see Case study 3).

Box 14.5 is a case study of a patient who presented with acute anxiety alongside existential anxiety.

Hypnotherapy interventions were used:

- To induce relaxation and use a dial to reduce her anxiety
- To slow her breathing and teach diaphragmatic breathing
- For accessing a safe place
- The anaesthetic glove technique was used in order to reduce the pain in her chest area.

The following approaches worked well for Julie: by inducing relaxation and offering her an opportunity to find a dial, which she could turn down in order to reduce her anxiety levels, helped to reverse the fight-or-flight mechanism. Through making her aware that she had adopted a 'brace position' allowed her to change her stance. This reduced the chest pain along with the subsequent fear of a heart attack. Slowing her breathing down and

---

BOX 14.5 Case study 3

Julie, aged 39 years, with oesophageal cancer and secondary disease in her chest wall, presented as being very anxious. She reported a number of symptoms including: difficulty sleeping, inability to relax, and feelings of panic with hyperventilation and chest pains. The chest pains had been investigated several times and no physiological abnormalities were identified. Her anxieties included: fear of dying from either the cancer or cardiac symptoms and feeling out of control. Julie's fight-or-flight mechanism had been triggered on receiving the news about her secondary cancer. Since then she had adopted a protective 'bracing' posture, which was possibly a subconscious way of protecting herself from impending danger. This was contributing to her chest pains and the psychological fear attached to the chest pains brought about a vicious circle of pain and fear.

teaching her to imagine that she was filling up a balloon at her abdomen as she breathed in, taught her to use diaphragmatic breathing.

Accessing a safe place increased her sense of security. It also reduced her sense of isolation by inviting her to have a companion in her safe place. She was able to use this place when she was having her treatment. The 'glove anaesthesia' approach entailed asking Jane to put her hand into an anaesthetic glove and move the glove onto the painful area of her chest. Yapko (2003: 362) suggests that in this approach 'the sensation of numbness encourages the change in perception of temperature, that is, the coolness of the hand'.

ADJUSTMENT

Each patient's response to his or her illness is unique, and therefore helping them through the anxiety of adjustment, requires an individualized holistic approach. If patients fail to adjust, either due to the overwhelming nature of the situation, or because of inadequate coping strategies, this can result in them being diagnosed with an adjustment disorder. Patients need to adjust to the trauma(s), which relate to the disease or subsequent treatments. This can be on many levels from physical, psychological, emotional, social and existential. In order to adjust this requires the person to work through the stages described by the seminal research of Kubler-Ross (1969) and Weisman and Worden (1976). These studies give a useful framework to identify stages that patients may be experiencing, although the sequence these take will vary from person to person. The initial stages of shock, numbness and denial are a way of coping psychologically and techniques aimed at bringing the knowledge into awareness too soon should be avoided. However, once this stage has passed, or if denial is proving to be problematic, then accessing information from the unconscious can help the process of adjustment.

WORKING WITH THE PERSON'S VIEW OF THEIR ILLNESS

How the person sees himself or herself and how they view their illness are important areas to assess. Speigal (1993) suggests that by asking patients to describe their illness gives an insight into their lives, as he sees illness as being symbolic of life's dilemmas. The illness is often described in many ways and the language patients use gives us a wealth of information to work with when using hypnotherapy techniques. It is important to note, however, that not all patients who are willing to describe their illness either metaphorically or in images, will go on to work with these.

For those patients who want to work in this way, information can be elicited and worked on through a number of approaches. Examples are: by encouraging patients to write down, or tell their narrative, draw their cancer, or how they view themselves, how they see their journey and what it feels like to be on this journey. Working with the images and words used, especially the negative ones can help the patient regain control over the situation. It also helps them to attach personal meaning to it, which in itself can be very healing.

METAPHOR

Metaphors are an alternative way of describing something and working with metaphors is seen as a way of describing a certain situation or experience. Patients often use metaphors to describe their experiences, as it has a way of distancing them psychologically from the enormity of the situation. It is also a rich and colourful way of letting another person know what that experience is like. When patients use metaphors to describe their experiences, these are opportunities not to be missed by the therapist and an introduction into their meaning is to reflect them back and inquire what they mean to the patient. Patients often use powerful metaphors such as 'being on a roller coaster' or 'feeling like they are drowning', 'cut adrift' and many more. In trance, the therapist can help to change the images attached to these metaphors, resulting in the patient feeling much more in control. However, before working in trance it is useful to elicit what positive outcome the patient would like to achieve in relation to the metaphor.

Disease metaphors

Disease metaphors are very important and through eliciting the meaning attached to them and how this links to the patient's life can be very empowering. Disease can be seen in many ways; such as invasive, or a punishment, or strangling. Helping the person to live with advancing disease through using hypnotherapy techniques can bring about a change on many levels for the patient. It is important to find out whether the disease metaphor is external or internal to the person and work towards transforming the negative image/metaphor. One way of explaining this is they are no longer at war with the disease or their body and have learned a way of adjusting.

Common illness metaphors often include a journey. Patients can talk about their illness as a metaphorical journey or their dreams may involve a journey. Again this can lend itself to hypnotherapy techniques by exploring the journey and working with the patient to make positive changes, which their unconscious knows is right for them. Kearney (1997) describes his work with a terminally ill young man who was anxious about his illness, but who never openly discussed it. However, through working with the image of a journey where he was on a boat with either someone he knew or someone he knew being at the destination (the companion). As part of the therapy he was able to metaphorically begin the process of separation from his family, who were on a liner going in the opposite direction.

ADJUSTING TO COPE WITH A MORTAL WOUND

Michael Kearney (1997, 2000) a palliative care consultant offers examples of how to work with patients in order to heal their mortal wounds. He reminds us is that helping some people to adjust will require a paradigm shift. This means that where we cannot change the situation (such as where death is imminent, or deformities are permanent), we need to help the patient to change how they view the situation. When this does not occur, patients exhibit symptoms of anxiety or depression. Kearney (1997) suggests that if we fail to do this, we are staying with them in their struggle and failing to give them the choice of a way out of the struggle. Sometimes this can mean helping them to find a way of re-framing a situation, while at other times it means helping them to accept the inevitability of their impending death.

On completion of the imagework, I checked out with Jane what she was experiencing. I used Kearney's (1997) advice and avoided using interpretation, but placed the value on the interaction between the conscious and unconscious mind. Jane reported feeling much freer following the imagery. In a following session, we worked on a distressing dream, which Jane had experienced, in which a black cloak was trying to engulf her and she was calling for help, but no one was there. Again avoiding any direct interpretation to her imminent death we worked with the feelings, which the dream evoked, which were of isolation and lacking support. Together we looked at what support she needed now her disease was advancing and how she might get support and from whom this would be.

In his work, Kearney (1997) talks about patients needing to adopt both the heroic stance but also experience a metaphorical descent, which is essential at different times in the illness. For Jane the heroic stance was important at the beginning of her illness and throughout her treatment. However, the time came when she had to consider a different stance. This initially left Jane feeling out of control and the need to regain control was important for her. The healing came when Jane acknowledged that she could not control what would happen in relation to how her illness progressed. However, what she could control was how she responded to it.

Viktor Frankl (1987) a Jewish psychiatrist and survivor of Auschwitz is well qualified to understand this position. He reminds us that:

Everything can be taken from man but one thing can't, and that is to choose one's attitude in any given set of circumstances, to choose one's own way.

DREAMS

When people are experiencing existential crises it is not uncommon for them to experience both waking and sleeping dreams. Marie Louise von Franz (in Kearney 1997) suggests 'nature, through dreams, prepares us for death. Dreams contain messages and symbols which are all an expression of self' and as such have the answer to patient's existential concerns. The ability to work with dreams offers the therapist a rich source of information, which may not need interpreting, and can therefore bypass cognitions.

Encouraging the patient to keep a dream diary or to draw their dreams gives the therapist an opportunity to work with them. Dreams like metaphors can be worked with and changed until they provide the ending, which the person's unconscious is comfortable with. Examples include: deathbed scenes where the images of family members can be changed, anxiety-provoking situations, which are symbolic of their cancer journey, can be altered through using empathic understanding. Patients often report images of their own funeral and this may relate to anticipatory grieving for their own death. Although this is uncomfortable for the patient, it can be even more distressing if therapists are unwilling to go with them to this place. Just by normalizing and validating this existential experience allows the person to know, that this image, although unpleasant, is preparing them psychologically for their own impending death.

Finally, therapists need to heed Kearney's advice in relation to helping patients adjust to this situation. He suggests that it is important for us to remember, 'no matter how skilled or humane our care of the dying is, it does not, and cannot make it all better'. He adds that, 'It's not alright and no matter what we might do to make it easier, death remains the ultimate separation, the ultimate unknown' (Kearney 1997: 23).

CONCLUSION

Existential anxiety is a common problem for patients who are facing their own mortality due to a life-threatening illness. For a therapist to be a companion on the patient's existential journey requires self-awareness and a well-developed therapeutic relationship. Working with the soul while using various hypnotherapy techniques will help the person adjust to their impending death.

REFERENCES

Barraclough, J., 1999. Cancer and emotion, a practical guide to psycho-oncology, second ed. Wiley, Chichester.

Bion, W.R., 1962. A psycho-analytic theory of thinking. Int. J. Psychoanal. 43 (Parts 4–5), 306–310.

Campbell, A., 1994. Moderated love: a theology of professional care. SPCK, London.

Cassell, E., 1991. The nature of suffering and the goals of medicine. Oxford University Press, Oxford.

Cassidy, S., 1988. Sharing the darkness: the spirituality of caring. Darton, London.

Cawthorn, A., 2006. Working with the denied body. In: Mackereth, P.A., Carter, A. (Eds.), Massage and bodywork: adapting therapies for cancer care. Churchill Livingstone, Edinburgh.

Clarkson, P., 1992. Transactional analysis psychotherapy an integrated approach. Routledge, London.

Cunningham, A.J., 2000. The healing journey: overcoming the crisis of cancer. Key Porter Books, Toronto.

Davis Brigham, D., 1996. Imagery for getting well, clinical applications of behavioural medicine. Norton, New York.

Deurzen-Smith, V., 1988. Existential counseling in practice. Sage, London.

Deurzen-Smith, V., 1995. Existential therapy. Regent's College, London.

Erskine, R.G., Moursund, P., Trautmann, R.J., 1999. Beyond empathy: a therapy of contact-in relationship. Edwards Brothers, Michigan.

Frankl, V.E., 1987. Man's search for meaning: an introduction to logotherapy. Hodder and Stoughton, New York.

Fishback Powers, M., 1993. Footprints. Marshall Pickering, London.

Heidegger, M., 1927. Being and time (J. Macquarrie, E.S. Robinson, 1962, Trans.). Harper & Row, London.

Honderich, T., 1995. The Oxford companion to philosophy. Oxford University Press, Oxford.

Inwood, M., 1997. Heidegger: a very short introduction. Oxford University Press, Oxford.

Johns, C., 2004. Being mindful, easing suffering. Jessica Kingsley, London.

Kearney, M., 1997. Mortally wounded: stories of soul pain, death and healing. Touchstone, New York.

Kearney, M., 2000. A place of healing: working with suffering in living and dying. Oxford University Press, Oxford.

Kierkegaard, S., 1844. The concept of anxiety (R. Thote, 1980, Trans.). Princeton University Press, Princeton, NJ.

King, M.E., Citrenbaum, C.M., 1993. Existential hypnotherapy. Guildford Press, London.

Kubler-Ross, E., 1969. On death and dying. Tavistock, London.

Kubler-Ross, E., 1997. The wheel of life. Scribner, New York.

Leuner, H., 1969. Guided affective imagery (GAI). A method of intensive psychotherapy. Am. J. Psychother. 23 (1), 4–21.

Mindell, A., 2003. Metaskills: the spiritual art of therapy, second ed. Lao Tse Press, Portland.

Narayanasamy, A., 1996. Spiritual care of chronically ill patients. Br. J. Nurs. 5 (7), 411–416.

Neimeyer, R.A., 1994. Death anxiety handbook: research, instrumentation and application. Taylor & Francis, Washington, DC.

NICE (National Institute for Clinical Excellence), 2004. Improving supportive and palliative care for adults with cancer: the manual. NICE, London.

Rinpoche, S., 1998. The Tibetan book of living and dying. HarperCollins, San Francisco.

Saunders, C., 1995. Hastings Cent. Rep. 25 (3), 44–45.

Seigal, B.S., 2001. Peace, love and healing. Quill, New York.

Speigal, D., 1993. Living beyond limits: new hope and help facing life threatening illness. Random House, New York.

Spinelli, E., 1989. The interpreted world: an introduction to phenomenological psychology. Sage, London.

Walter, T., 1997. The ideology and organization of spiritual care: three approaches. Palliat. Med. 1, 21–30.

Weisman, A.D., Worden, J.W., 1976. The existential plight in cancer: significance of the first 100 days. Int. J. Psychiatry Med. 7 (1), 1–15.

Wells, M., 2001. The impact of cancer. In: Corner, J., Bailey, C. (Eds.), Cancer nursing: care in context. Blackwell Science, Iowa.

Yapko, M.D., 2001. Treating depression with hypnosis integrating cognitive–behavioural and strategic approaches. Brunner Routledge, Florence.

Yapko, M.D., 2003. Trancework. An introduction to the practice of clinical hypnosis, third ed. Brunner/Routledge, New York.

Existential hypnotherapy in life-threatening illness

INDEX

Note: Page numbers followed by *b* indicate boxes, *f* indicate figures and *t* indicate tables.

emotional release and safe therapeutic practice, 122–123

evidence for change in mental states, 117–118

hypnotic trance incorporation in, 115–128

questions for carer/patient staff, 125

questions for therapist, 124–125

trance state and, 122–123, 122*b*

use of, 34

training *see* education and training

trance *see* hypnosis

transpersonal relationship, 223

trauma, body image, 144–146

travelling companion, 68–69

trespass against the person ('battery'), 35–36

U

UK Confederation of Hynotherapy Organizations, 42

Uncovered Relationship, 223*b*

unprofesional practice, reporting, 41

utilization approach, 68

V

vein enlargment, cancer and, 176

vessel approach to hypnosis, 187

visual analogue scale (VAS), 172–173

visualization, 4, 21

vulnerable adults, 37

W

Wanting Relationship, 223*b*

weight control, 136–137

willpower, 154

World Health Organization Quality of Life Scale (WHOQoL), 86

wound healing, 11

INDEX

Printed in the United States
By Bookmasters